Progression

Progression

A FEMALE ADOLESCENTS' AND PARENTS' GUIDE TO GYNECOLOGIC HEALTH

Dr. Shamanique Bodie-Williams

This book is meant to serve as a guide. It is not intended to provide clinical advice, therapy, counseling, or take the place of your health-care provider. You are advised to discuss health issues with your health-care provider. Neither the publisher nor the author take responsibility for any possible consequences resulting from treatment, action, or application of information recommended by this book to the reader.

ISBN-13: 978-0-9600911-0-2

Editors: Sharanna Bodie, Ally Carlton-Smith

Table of Contents

Acknowledgments

THANK YOU, LORD, FOR THE spiritual insight and wisdom to write this book.

Thank you, Wellington, for your ongoing support and encouragement.

Lluvia, thank you for helping me to see things through your life. Thank you for giving me a teenager's point of view.

Anita and Carlton Bodie, if I could only bottle you. I can only imagine what the world would be like if there were more parents like you. You sacrificed day in and day out so that we could have the best education. You showed us everyday not only how to live but how to thrive. We learned how to treat others well by watching the examples you set. To God be the glory for you!

Valdez, McCain, and Sharanna, thank you for being the best siblings a person could desire. Thank you for your continual encouragement and support. I love you all. Sharanna, thank you for taking the time to read through my manuscript and give your input.

Thank you to my well-wishers in the Grand Bahama Health Services. Thank you to the medical students and house officers that I have the honor of working with on a daily basis who continue to inspire me and allow me to discuss my book and research ideas with them. Dr Bowe, thank you for reading through my manuscript and giving your opinion.

In Loving Memory of:
Dr. Katrice Maycock, January 17th, 1988 - August 4th, 2019
My mentee. You made the difference everyday.

Dr. Augustine Ohueyi, August 18th, 1966 - October 30th, 2019

My colleague and a friend. A giant loss to the patients and healthcare system of The Bahamas.

Revelation 21:4 King James Version (KJV)
And God shall wipe away all tears from their eyes; and there shall be no more death, neither sorrow, nor crying, neither shall there be any more pain: for the former things are passed away.

Scriptures are also taken from The Holy Bible, The King James Version (KJV)

Introduction

❧

IN MY PRACTICE, I TAKE care of patients of different ages. To date, the age range of my patients has been from less than a year old to ninety-eight years old. Some may say "from the toothless to the toothless." Like other obstetrician-gynecologists, I care for quite a few adolescents and young adult ladies. I am a physician who specializes in women's health. But, I have been a teenager and I have a teenage daughter. With that in mind, I can see the issues from different perspectives. I wanted to create this guide to help teenagers and their parents/guardians navigate the complexities of the female reproductive health system.

Studies show that adolescents could be at risk for possibly life-threatening health issues. I know that part of decreasing that risk is education. In the following pages, I hope to share some information on common issues and some not so common issues. This book is in no way meant to substitute for consultation and care by your medical care provider, but it is meant to be a starting point for information.

This book was born out of my passion for caring for you. It is my desire to see you progress. I want you to live your very best life. Your life can be impacted by decisions and experiences that happen on a day-to-day basis.

Jeremiah 29:11 (KJV)
For I know the thoughts that I think toward you, saith the Lord, thoughts of peace, and not evil, to give you an expected end."

CHAPTER 1

What Is Puberty?
What Is Adolescence?

⚬⚬⚬

BY NOW, YOU'VE PROBABLY HAD a health science class in school. You may have gone through all this already. The students in your health class may have been different genders or the same gender. Either way, it may have been an uncomfortable topic that you wanted to skip. So, let us consider this a review—your review. This time, it is all about you! It is about your body, the changes that are happening within you, and concerns that you may have.

The reproductive system that you were born with changes as you grow older. Before this stage, you probably noticed that boys and girls have similar parts on the top. You may have gone to the pool, lake, or beach together. You may not have worn a swim top. No big deal. But somewhere you started to change. This change happens over time and is called puberty.

Some of you like the changes that are happening. You may look forward to them. Others may not be happy about them at all. I remember sneaking into my mom's drawer as a young girl to try on her black satin bra. I would go into her closet and pull out her heels and purses and try them out too. At the time, neither the shoes nor the bra fit me. I wondered about that time to come when they would. I wanted to have more than just a flat chest. I wanted to wear a bra and heels. Eventually, changes happened to my body, too. Now I can wear a bra and heels.

PUBERTY

Puberty is the process that boys and girls go through to become sexually mature adults. It is the period from childhood to adulthood. The start of puberty is different for everyone. Puberty usually occurs in girls between the ages of eight and sixteen, while in boys it generally occurs later. Most girls start to notice changes in their bodies between the ages of ten and fourteen, which continue over a number of years.

The body makes chemicals called *hormones* that start and control these changes. Puberty involves physical changes such as the development of secondary sex characteristics. These are the physical features associated with females (such as the growth of pubic hair, breasts, acne, changes in height, etc.).

The physical changes are only part of the picture. Your thoughts and emotions will change too. Your ability to think about ideas and situations improves. You try to figure out who you are in your friends' eyes, your parents' eyes, and your own eyes. You may try to "fit in" or decide not to try to "fit in."

An important part of puberty is that you are able to integrate bodily changes into your self-identity (who you think you are) and to incorporate others' responses to these changes into that self-identity. In other words, taking what is happening to your body, what is happening in your mind, and how other people act toward you and putting it all together. That is *a lot* to deal with. You may feel happy one moment or sad and confused the next.

During the early stages of puberty, your friendships between same sex peers may become more important. This may happen because you are going through similar changes and you may feel that they can relate to you more. You may have similar changes in your appearance and your thinking. But sometimes you may not identify with your same sex peers. You may feel that you have nothing in common with them and that you cannot relate to each other.

Your body is changing physically and you have new and complicated emotions. You also have to deal with your own changes, your friends' changes, and your relationship with your parents/guardians. Go figure. It may be overwhelming.

ADOLESCENCE
Adolescence includes persons in the age group of ten to nineteen. It also includes early adolescence (ages thirteen to fourteen), middle adolescence (ages fifteen to seventeen) and late adolescence (eighteen to nineteen). This period includes growth, development, and increased pressures, and is generally the time when you start to discover who you are. This is considered a period of change or transition. There is probably no other time in life when you are going to change as much and in such a short time. Each person changes differently. This change is affected by the culture that you are in (also known as your environment). For example, the experience of a young lady growing up in The Bahamas may be different from one growing up in the United States or India. This phase of life establishes the foundation for your growth and development in your life to come.

YOUNG ADULTS
This includes persons from ten to twenty-four years old. This period can overlap with adolescence. This part of development is key. You mature and change during this time and your brain continues to develop.

SUMMARY POINTS

* You and your needs require attention.
* No two adolescents or young adults are the same.
* It is important for you to understand the changes that are happening to you at this time.
* Decisions made during this stage can affect you now and possibly later.

Ezekiel 16: 7 New International Version (NIV)
I made you grow like a plant of the field. You grew and developed and entered puberty. Your breasts had formed and your hair had grown, yet you were stark naked.

CHAPTER 2

First Ever Visit to the Gynecologist

❦

Jeremiah 33:6 (NIV)
Nevertheless, I will bring health and healing to it; I will heal my people and will let them enjoy abundant peace and security.

I enter the room to greet my next patient of the day. My next patient is you. It is your first visit that is not with a pediatrician. Sometimes when I enter the room you are texting. Sometimes you look defiant, upset that your guardian has made you come. Sometimes you look bored. Sometimes you are apprehensive. But, sometimes you are excited. You have questions that you are eager to have answered. You may or may not want to be here—you have not quite made up your mind. You want to know what to expect and why you are here. Whatever emotion you're experiencing, I have probably encountered it before and it is okay. I see your mom (sister, aunt, grandmother) sitting in the corner. She is glad that she brought you to the doctor. She too has a wealth of emotions and expectations. Although she may not know what to expect, she has brought you because she understands the importance of preventative health care.

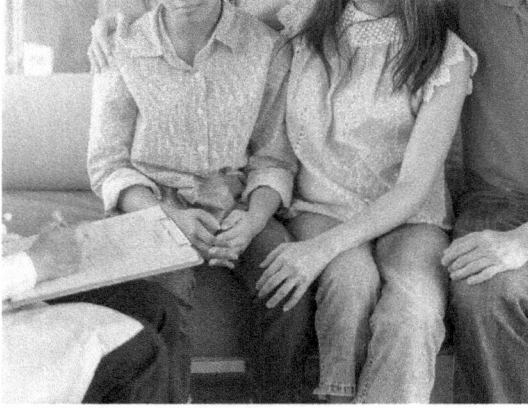

In the following pages, I will arm you with information to help you make the most out of your visit to the doctor. This may be a female doctor, such as a gynecologist. But you may also see another health-care provider such as a family practitioner, a physician assistant, or a nurse practitioner. I want you to have an idea of what will happen when you go for that first visit.

The first female well-visit shapes how you look at future medical visits. I still remember the first time I went to see a gynecologist. A good experience during this visit goes a long way in helping to build a good relationship with your doctor. It may improve your lifestyle choices. It may encourage you to address health problems and seek treatment early. Your visits may provide education about the benefits of preventive care and address your issues and needs.

WHEN TO SEE A GYNECOLOGIST

It is a good idea to see a gynecologist once your period starts or even before. A good time to consider the initial visit is between the ages of thirteen to fifteen. This enables your gynecologist to talk about what is normal and what is not normal. If you have a problem at a younger age, your pediatrician or family doctor may refer you to a gynecologist or a pediatric gynecologist (a doctor who specializes in problems in younger age groups).

PATIENT FORM

You may have been asked to fill out forms online before the visit or at the start of the visit. The information on these forms can give the health-care provider information on how best to help you. The questionnaire may have questions that ask about your family and any medical problems that are in the family. There are usually questions about your medical history, medications, your allergies to medicines or foods, and about any operations you may have had.

SCREENING

The medical provider may have an assistant who might ask you some basic questions. They will measure your weight, height, blood pressure, heart rate, breathing rate, and temperature. They may send you to the bathroom to leave a urine sample in a container. They may take a look at your urine and check it for sugar, protein, your hydration status, or for signs of infection.

LET'S TALK

After you have been greeted, the health care provider may sit with you and your guardian and review all the information that was written down. This is a good time to ask any questions that you may have and see how comfortable you feel. Practitioners are increasingly busy; I advise thinking about the questions or topics that you want to address before your visit. You may even consider writing them down.

EXAMINATION

This involves checking you out to make sure that parts of your body are where they would normally be and to make sure that those that are there are normal.

- Your skin will be inspected.
- Your thyroid (a gland in the neck) may be examined.
- Your breasts may be examined, and you may be taught how to check your own breasts for any abnormalities.
- The pelvic area may be examined. A speculum exam (a device that allows the health care provider to inspect the lining of the vagina and the neck of the womb, which is located at the top of the vagina) may or may not be done.
- A biannual exam (an exam where health-care providers use a finger or fingers to palpate the cervix, uterus, and ovaries) is not always done as it depends on the problem/complaint and the clinician).
- Your heart and lungs may be listened to with a stethoscope.
- Other parts of your body may be examined if needed.

Each health care provider has a different approach to how they examine a patient. When I do an examination, I always ask for your permission or consent. I will take the time to explain what I am doing and why. I will give you information about the body part that I am examining and the findings. I will also explain how to check the body part yourself if it is one that you can check. For example, I will teach you how to do a breast self-exam.

LABORATORY TESTS

These may be ordered depending on your age group. For example, the doctor may check your complete blood count (CBC) to make sure your blood count is not low (anemia) or may check your glucose (sugar level).

CONCLUSION OF VISIT

After the visit, the doctor may give you a summary of the findings and review any topics that were talked about at the start of the visit.

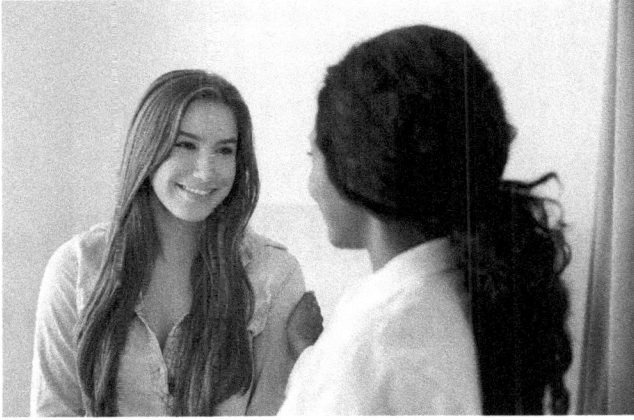

SUMMARY POINTS

* To make the most of your visit, take some time in advance to create a list of questions and concerns.
* Your visit is an important opportunity for you and your doctor to get to know each other.
* You may have to fill out a form.
* You may be screened. Information like weight, height, and blood pressure may be measured.
* You may be seen and examined by the doctor.
* Your health-care provider may order blood work.
* Get your health-care provider's contact details so that you have the chance to address any questions or concerns that may come up after the visit.

CHAPTER 3

The Parts of Your Body and Some Other Stuff

~⨂~

Psalm 139:14 (KJV)
I will praise thee; for I am fearfully and wonderfully made: marvelous are thy works; and that my soul knoweth right well.

The parts of the body are like snowflakes. No two parts are the same. They may have the same function, but it is important to understand that they are different. Your parts are yours and yours alone! They may look similar to your mom's, your aunt's, or your friends', but they may not actually be so. They are uniquely yours. I ask you to not use what you may find in magazines or on the Internet as the standard of normal. Resist the temptation to compare your body parts with other young ladies.

Female external reproductive organs

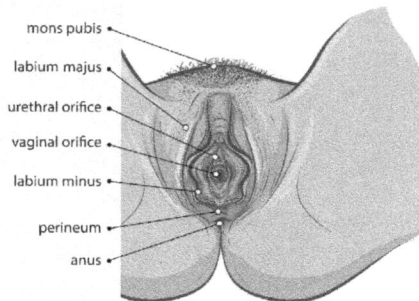

Figure 1. Female external reproductive organs

Everyone is different. If you have concerns or are not sure, go through these questions with a qualified health-care provider. They can do an exam and let you know if there is something that is not normal. The parts of the body are what we call anatomy. Some parts of the female system are internal (inside the body), and some parts of the female system are external (outside the body).

Vulva — The vulva includes the parts that make up the female external (outside) genitalia

These include the:

* Mons pubis
* Labia majora
* Labia minora
* Clitoris
* Vestibule
* Bartholin's glands

Labia Majora — Two flaps of skin on the side of the vaginal opening. These can vary in size, shape, and color. On the top they come together to form the mons pubis. They have hair follicles (terminal hair) and sweat glands.

Labia Minora — Two flaps of skin that are on the inside of the labia majora. These can vary in size, shape, and color. They do not have any hair. They come together at the top and join around the clitoris

Clitoris —This is an organ located at the top of the vulva. Part of it can be seen if you look on the outside of the vulva and part of it cannot be seen. It may be as small as a pea or as big as a thumb. It has tons of nerve endings that are for sexual function (later in life).

Bartholin's Glands (Greater Vestibular Glands) —These are two pea-sized glands that are located near the opening of the vagina on the left and the right. These glands make secretions such as mucous. If they get blocked, this area may swell.

The Skene's Gland (Lesser Vestibular Glands) — These are on either side of the opening for the urethra. They can release secretions.

Perineum — This is the mostly flat area that is under the labia majora and above the anus. It has a perineal body that is made of muscles that support the vagina and come together in this area.

Vestibule — When you separate the labia minora, the area that is seen is the vestibule. This is where the urethra and the Skene's glands are located.

Urethra — This is the passageway for urine (pee) to leave the body. You can think of it as a tunnel or tube-like structure. It is located above the entrance to the vagina.

Vagina and Hymen — This is a highway or passageway to your reproductive system. It connects the outside to the inside. It allows your period to pass from the womb to the outside of the body. The vagina increases in length as you get older. The vagina has secretions that may come out, depending on your hormones The vagina has a hymen (a seal) that usually stays in place until a person becomes sexually active, in most cases. The hymen has different shapes. It normally allows the menstrual blood to flow through it.

Anus (Butthole) — This is the opening at the end of your digestive system that takes waste out of the body.

FEMALE REPRODUCTIVE SYSTEM

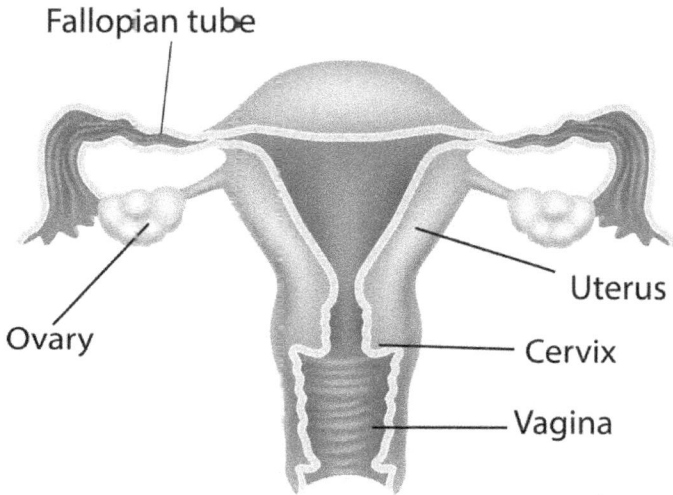

Figure 2. Internal female reproductive organs

Uterus — This is a pear-shaped organ that is made up of muscle. It is broken into three parts: the body, the lower uterine segment, and the cervix. The uterus lining (endometrium) breaks off (sheds) when you menstruate (have a period). The lower end of the uterus is connected to the vagina by the cervix. The upper part of the uterus is connected to the fallopian tubes. The uterus is also responsible for holding any future pregnancies you may have.

Cervix — This is the neck of the womb and the lower part of the uterus. To give you an idea of what the cervix looks like, think of a pink dough-nut and imagine the center was the size of a pen tip. The cervix has an outer portion and inner portion that look like this modified donut center. This passageway is the route that the menses (period) takes to leave the uterus. The cervix has a portion than can be seen when we do a speculum exam. Feel the tip of your nose. This is usually what a normal cervix in someone of your age group will feel like.

Ovaries — These are organs that produce and release eggs (oocytes). The size of the ovaries changes with age. In adolescence, they may be the size of a grape and have the appearance of chewed bubble gum. They make hormones such as estrogen and progesterone, and the ovaries play a role in the control of your period.

Fallopian Tubes —These are narrow tubes that guide the egg to the womb during ovulation (the period when you release an egg). Think of these tubes like a highway for the egg to travel on. The fallopian tube.

Glands — These are organs that make and release substances such as hormones (which are responsible for actions in other organs) to perform a specific role or function in the body. Some glands release substances directly into the bloodstream. The main glands involved in menstrual cycle regulation are as follows:

* Hypothalamus
* Pituitary
* Thyroid

Thyroid — This gland in the front of the neck makes hormones that control metabolism (the way your body burns energy).

Hypothalamus — This gland makes several hormones that start and stop the production of different hormones that control the function of other glands. Consider it a "boss" gland. It sends messages/signals to the pituitary gland and is located close to the pituitary gland.

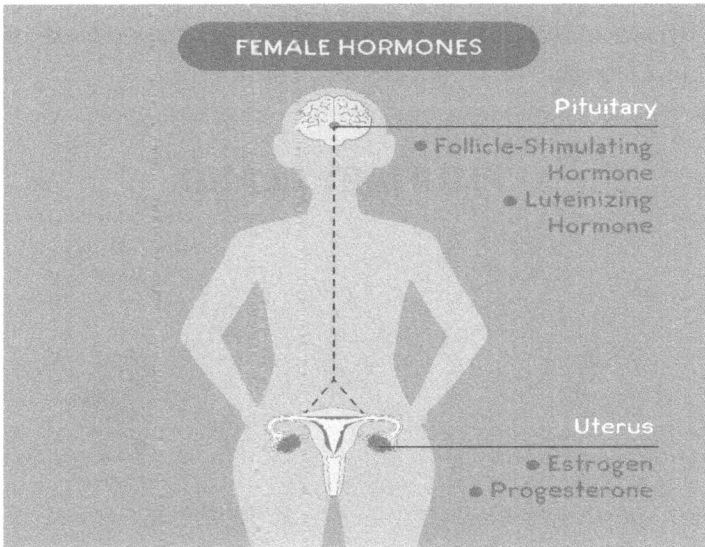

Figure 3. Female hormones

Pituitary Gland — This pea-sized gland has two parts (anterior and posterior) and is found at the base of the brain. It is like a parent gland, as it makes many hormones that travel throughout the body to control other glands such as the thyroid and ovaries. The hormones made by the pituitary gland that we need to know about in regard to menstruation are as follows:

ANTERIOR (FRONT) LOBE

* Adrenocorticotropic hormone (ACTH) – Causes cortisol to be made in the adrenal gland.
* Follicle-stimulating hormone (FSH) – Stimulates maturity of the ovum (egg).
* Growth hormone (GH) – Causes the release of hormones involved in your growth.
* Luteinizing hormone (LH) – Cause the ovaries to release hormones and triggers ovulation.

* Thyroid stimulating hormone (TSH) – Causes release of the thyroid hormone
* prolactin which causes production of breast milk.

PITUITARY GLAND

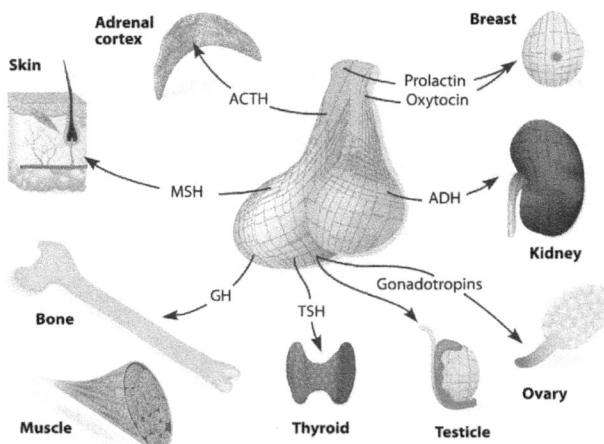

Figure 4. The hormones the pituitary gland make and the parts that they work on

SUMMARY POINTS

* We all have body parts that are different.
* You have parts that are on the outside such as the vulva, urethra, and vaginal opening.
* You have parts on the inside such as the vagina, cervix, uterus, fallopian tubes, and ovaries.
* The occurrence of the menstrual cycle is controlled by hormones that released from glands such as the hypothalamus, the thyroid, and the pituitary gland.

CHAPTER 4

Where Are the Breasts Going?

❦

SONG OF SOLOMON 7:7 (NIV)

Your stature is like that of the palm, and your breasts like clusters of fruit.

If you are under twenty and reading this and you look at your body parts today, they are not going to look the same six months to a year from now. Just like your journey through this life, they have a journey too; and that journey takes time. The following is meant to serve as a guide to help you understand where your parts are and where they are going.

BREAST DEVELOPMENT

The breast bud is one of the first signs of puberty. When your ovaries start to make hormones, the fat in your breast begins to increase. Yes, the breast has fat tissue. The growth of your breasts begins with the formation of secretory glands at the end of the milk ducts. The breasts and duct system continue to grow and mature with the development of many glands and lobules.

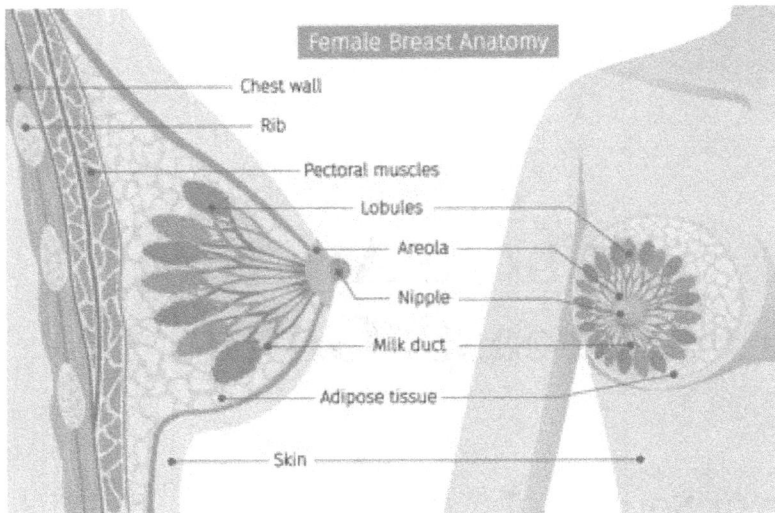

Figure 5. The anatomy of the female breast

The speed at which breasts grow is different for everyone, but the stages are the same. Breast development occurs in five stages.

Table 1

Staging for Breast Development (Tanner Staging)	
Stage One:	In preadolescence, the breasts are flat. The tip of the nipple is raised.
Stage Two	Buds come, breast and nipple fat begins to form, and the dark area of skin around the nipple gets bigger.
Stage Three	Breasts are slightly larger with a different type of breast tissue (glandular breast tissue) present. Your breasts may be shaped like a cone first and then they become rounder. The areola starts to darken.
Stage Four	The nipple and areola (dark area around the nipple) become raised and form a second mound above the rest of the breast.
Stage Five	Mature adult breasts are rounded and only the nipple is raised. Full adult size has been achieved

Breast development may take three to five years, but for some girls it may take longer. Each month, changes in hormones happen. Estrogen causes the growth of milk ducts in the breasts. Progesterone is the boss of the second half of the cycle. It stimulates the formation of the milk glands. These hormones play a part in changes such as increase in size, swelling, and tenderness. Most young ladies will have some breast development by fifteen or sixteen years old.

As your breasts develop, you may become self-conscious of your nipples showing through your clothes, or you may need more supportive clothing. Some options would be to wear:

* A T-shirt or tank top under your clothes
* A camisole (undershirt with thin straps)
* Trainers
* A bra (soft cup, underwire, padded, sports, or cropped top)

DETERMINING BRA SIZE

To determine your bra size, you can:

* Estimate it
* Be fitted at a store
* Measure yourself

The bra size is made of the band number and a letter. For example, size 32 A

To get the band size, you would measure around your torso, just underneath your breasts. A 32 band size means that the measurement is 32 inches.

The letter refers to your cup (breast) size. It starts at AAA and goes up. To determine your cup size, you measure around the fullest part of your breasts and subtract that measurement from the first measurement. The difference between the two measurements would determine the cup size. So, if you are 32 A, the measurement of the breasts would be 33 inches and under the breasts would be 32 inches. That gives a difference of 1 inch.

Table 2

Bra Sizing Chart	
Inches Different	Size
1	A
2	B
3	C
4	D
5	DD
6	DDD & F

FEMALE BREAST SIZES

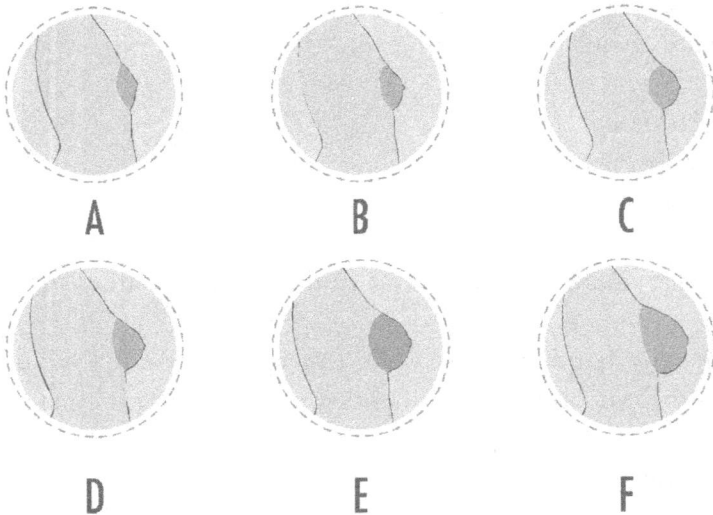

Figure 6. Female Breast Sizes

Finding the perfect fitting bra may take a few tries. Your perfect fit will change as your breasts change. Make sure your bra is not too tight. You should be able to get a finger between the bra band and your body. If your breasts are coming up over the top of the bra, then you need to go up a size. If the band is riding up in the back or your breast are falling out the bra, go down a band size.

ISSUES WITH THE BREASTS

Normal breast tissue can be lumpy and bumpy. Sometimes, you may not be sure what you are feeling. Trust how you feel. You can write down what you feel in the breast and where. Take note of when the concern started. If something doesn't feel right about your breast, let your doctor know. Below we will talk about some of the common breast concerns, such as breast pain, differences in how one breast looks compared to the other, nipple discharge, growth in the breast, and cancer.

BREAST PAIN (MASTALGIA)

Breast pain can be complicated. It may be related to the period (cyclic) or not related to the period (noncyclic). Pain can be in one breast or in both breasts. If it is cyclic pain, it usually goes away when the period ends.

If the pain is noncyclic (not related to the period), it could be caused by conditions that may affect the breast. such as adenomas, fibroadenomas, infection, or cancer. Or sometimes, you may feel pain in the breast that is actually caused by other body parts that are close to the breast. For example, inflammation of the chest muscles (costochondritis) or the joints can cause breast pain. At times, it may be caused by other issues, such as gallstones, causing inflammation inside of the body which then causes chest pain.

Breast pain can also be a side effect of medications such as birth control pills, antidepressants, blood pressure medications, and some heart medications. You also want to ensure your bra is fitting properly. With hormonal changes, the breast may become tender or sore before or during the menstrual cycle.

Diet changes such as decreasing caffeine intake, reducing your salt intake, and taking some vitamins such as Vitamin E, B6, B1, and Evening Primrose Oil may be helpful in reducing the pain. Exercise and maintaining a healthy weight may also decrease pain.

Wearing a supportive (sports) bra, keeping your stress level down, and taking over-the-counter pain medications, as directed, may be helpful. The good news is that many cases of breast pain go away with time, especially when related to the period. If you have breast pain, discuss this issue with your health-care provider who can examine you and help get to the root of the problem.

ASYMMETRY OF THE BREAST

The causes of asymmetry (when the size of one breast is different from the other) are not entirely known. This is usually not a cause for worry. However, it's a good idea to discuss this with your health-care provider. Consider using padded bras or bra pads to make the breasts appear more symmetrical. Once your breasts have completed development, you can revisit this issue with your doctor. Many are able to deal with it without surgical intervention, but if that is recommended, you may be referred to a plastic surgeon. If you have no breast tissue, this may point to a health condition that may need to be treated so that your breasts can develop normally.

ACCESSORY BREAST TISSUE

One to two out of one hundred ladies will have extra nipples or extra breast tissue. This may look like a breast with a nipple and areola or it may look like a lump under the skin. Accessory breast tissue is usually located below the normal breast tissue. You may not have any symptoms as a result of this or you may have pain or discharge. If you experience pain or discharge, you may choose to have the extra breast tissue removed. Discuss this with your health-care provider so that they can advise you or refer you to a physician who can remove the tissue.

DISORDERS OF THE FEMALE BREAST

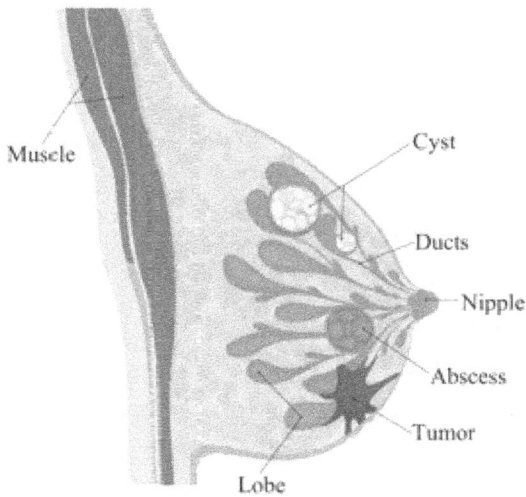

Figure 7. Disorders of the female breast

FIBROADENOMA

Fibroadenomas are the most common reason for breast lumps in your age group. They are non-cancerous (benign) firm lumps that may appear in the breast after puberty. Fibroadenomas are a result of overgrowth of connective tissue stroma of the breast. They are usually not painful. However, fibroadenomas may be tender, especially close to the period. This is more common in late adolescence. The growth may be rapid initially, and their average size is two to three centimeters. If you notice a lump in your breast, I recommend that you bring it to the attention of your health-care provider. Your health-care provider will use your medical history and a clinical exam to make the diagnosis. They may also confirm the findings with ultrasound.

FIBROCYSTIC BREAST CHANGES

These are noncancerous changes in the breast that are affected by your hormones. The breast fibers may form cysts, or there may be an increase in the connective tissue (fibrosis). These may change the way the breast feels upon examination. They may be painful, especially around your period or the time of ovulation. The breast may feel lumpy when examined and may improve once the period starts. Pain medication, vitamins, and lowering your caffeine intake may help decrease the pain. In some cases, birth control pills may also be used to help ease the pain.

BREAST CYSTS

A cyst is a sac filled with fluid. These can occur anywhere in the body, including the breasts. They can be in one or both breasts. You may be able to feel them in the breast and they may feel round and spongy. They may increase before your period and go away after. Sometimes they are large, tender, and cause pain. If this is the case, the cyst may be emptied of its contents (drained with a needle) and the fluid may be sent for additional testing.

NIPPLE DISCHARGE

This is usually a milky discharge that may be purulent (containing pus) or bloody. There are many different causes of breast discharge, including medications and mechanical causes, such as stimulation of the breast.

Milk production (galactorrhea) from the breast may happen if you are pregnant, postpartum, recently had a miscarriage, or are having a problem with the glands that produce hormones such as the thyroid or prolactin. The milk will usually come out of both breasts. Sometimes we are unable to find the reason why you are leaking milk from your breasts and the breast exam may be normal.

Purulent discharge is not normal. Usually it comes from one breast and may be caused by an infection, as discussed in the section on mastitis below. It may be different colors, such as grey, greenish, or bloody. Bloody discharge may be a result of fibrocystic changes, problems in the nipple, breast glands, or in the breast tissue. Two causes are intraductal papilloma and mammary duct ectasia

INTRADUCTAL PAPILLOMA

These are found in the ducts under the areola. Papilloma causes nipple discharge that may be bloody. They may be difficult to feel on exam. Imaging may help with the diagnosis. You may be referred to a breast specialist for additional management.

MAMMARY DUCT ECTASIA

This occurs when there is a blockage in the subareolar ducts and may result in discharge from the nipple. The discharge may be sticky and be different colors. The breast discharge will usually stop on its own. If it does not, your health-care provider may refer you to a surgeon to remove that area.

If you have discharge that persists, you should see your health-care provider. They may ask you to get testing and an ultrasound to try to determine why you are having the discharge.

MASTITIS AND BREAST ABSCESS

This is an infection of the breast that is mostly caused by common bacteria such as *Staphylococcus aureus*, group A *Streptococcus*, or *Enterococcus*. Your breasts may be tender, red, and warm. Your health-care provider may ask you to get an image of the breast called an ultrasound. Mastitis and breast abscesses are usually treated with a course of antibiotics. An abscess is a collection of pus (liquid produced by infected tissue, often yellow or green in appearance) that has accumulated in the body. In the case of an abscess, we may have to decrease the amount of infection by opening the area and draining it (incision and drainage).

PHYLLODES TUMORS

These are rare growths that may be cancerous or non-cancerous. In adolescents then tend to be non-cancerous. These tumors tend to grow rapidly and can come back or recur when removed.

BREAST CANCER OR BREAST METASTASIS

This is extremely rare in adolescents. If you have a family history of breast cancer, a personal history of breast cancer, or if you have had previous radiation exposure to the chest, this may increase your chance of getting breast cancer in adolescene. A breast metastasis is a cancer that starts in another part of the body and moves to the breast. If this is suspected, your provider may refer you for imaging. A sample of the problem area may be taken to make the diagnosis.

SUMMARY POINTS

* Breasts may not be there one day and then suddenly start to develop.
* Breast development happens in stages. They are changing and the development may take time.
* Your chest may hurt.
* The pain may or may not be related to the time of your period.
* You may now have to wear a bra.

- One of your breasts may be bigger than the other (asymmetry).
- You may have lumps and bumps in the breast.
- Most breast masses are non-cancerous.
- If you are concerned or if they do not go away, make sure you let your health-care provider know so that they can find out why and possibly make some recommendations.
- Ultrasound may be used along with an exam to make the diagnosis.

CHAPTER 5

Hair Is Here

❦

Luke 12:7 (KJV)
But even the very hairs of your head are all numbered. Fear not therefore: ye are of more value than many sparrows.

Hair everywhere—ugh! A few strands start in the pubic region and then under the arm. This is called pubarche and is caused by adrenarche.

Adrenarche, or the awakening of the adrenal glands, is the part of development where there is an increase in certain hormones that cause pubic hair, body odor, skin oiliness, and acne. Later, hair on the leg also increases. Hair then begins to grow down there—on the vulva—and increases throughout the years.

Hair has two types. Vellus hair is usually found on the face and chest and tends to be soft and fine. Terminal hair tends to be darker and coarser and is mostly found on your head, in your armpits, and in your vulvar area.

Table 3

Table for Pubic Hair Staging (Tanner Staging)	
Stage One	In preadolescence there is no pubic hair
Stage Two	Growth of long, slightly pigmented straight or curly hair along the labia
Stage Three	Hair is now darker and coarser. It spreads over the junction of the mons pubis.
Stage Four	The hair fills the entire area. It has not spread to the medial thighs.
Stage Five	Mature adult hair has spread to the medial surface of the thighs. This is adult pattern pubic hair.

This is one of the puberty changes that you may not like or you may not mind at all. You may choose to keep the hair well groomed, which may include trimming, shaving, waxing, using depilatory creams, or sugaring. It is important that you are comfortable with the decision. If you are doing any of the above and you are younger, discuss this with your parents. Take some time to read about the different methods.

Table 4

Temporary Methods of Hair Removal			
Method	*Advantages*	*Disadvantages*	*Duration (Average)*
Shaving—razor or electric (use of manual razor or electric blade)	Method is cheap and not painful.	May cause nicks and cuts. Effects do not last as long as some other methods.	1-3 days
Waxing	Effects last longer than shaving; it can be used for larger areas.	It may be more expensive and more painful than other methods.	4-6 weeks

Sugaring	It can be used for larger areas, effects may last longer and over time, may become permanent.	May be costly. More painful than trimming or shaving.	4-6 weeks
Chemical depilatories	Method is widely available. The effects last longer than shaving.	May contain possible skin irritants.	3-7 days
Trimming—cutting hair shorter with scissors	It is safe, cheap, and effective.	Not practical for large areas and some skin surfaces.	A few days
Tweezing	It is safe, cheap, and effective.	Not practical for large areas and some skin surfaces. It may be painful. Only used for small areas.	2-6 weeks

Suggestions for Methods of Removing Unwanted Hair

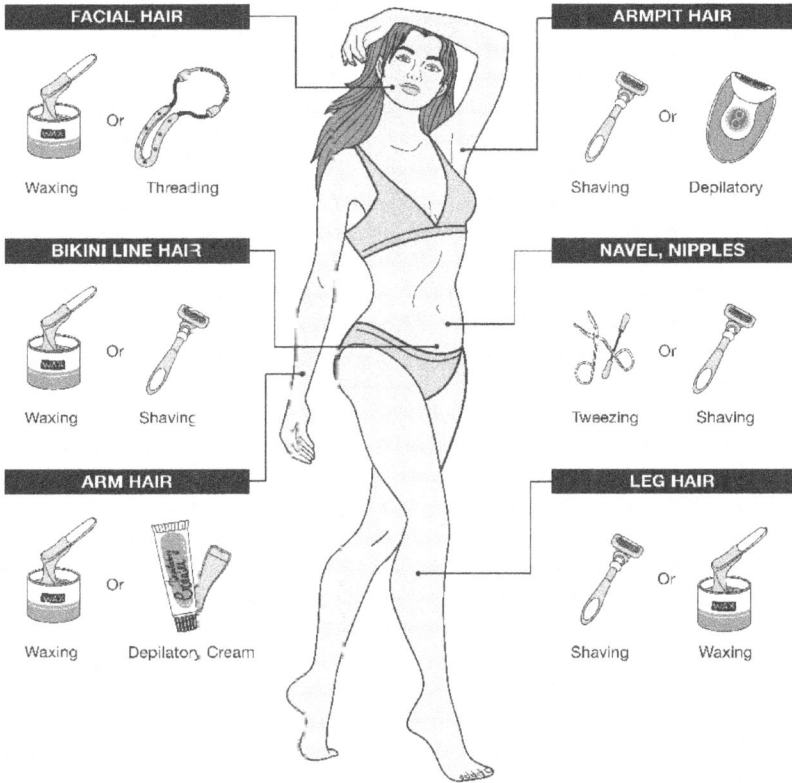

Figure 8. Tips for hair removal

Tips for Using Depilatory Creams and Lotions:

* Read the instructions. Do not leave on longer than advised.
* Check your skin type. For example, if you have sensitive skin, look for preparations intended for sensitive skin.
* Use a small amount on a small area first to ensure you do not have a reaction.

* Use the right type of depilatory on the right area—for example, legs for leg and bikini for the areas close to the vagina.
* Wipe the product off. Do not rub it into the skin.
* Make sure the hair is long enough so that the removal can work.
* If removal is not complete, wait before you reuse the product on the same area.

TIPS FOR SHAVING

* Never share a razor with another person, even a family member.
* Use a sharp, clean razor.
* Wet legs and use shaving cream.
* Take it slowly—you will most likely cut yourself at some point, but this will happen less and less with time.
* Apply only the needed pressure to the blade, being more careful around your bony parts such as the ankles and knees.
* Rinse your legs, check for cuts, and moisturize your skin after shaving.

I DON'T WANT TO REMOVE MY HAIR

If you want to leave your hair alone and that makes you more comfortable, that is okay, too. It is thought to be beneficial for those with sensitive skin to leave it alone. It is also thought that the hair may prevent body parts such as under the armpits from rubbing together. The vellus type of hair especially provides cushion and protection. If you choose to keep your hair, ensure that you keep the area clean to avoid the build up of bacteria and odors.

HAIR GROOMING

Remember to keep the hair on your head clean so that it does not smell. How often you wash your hair will depend on the type of hair you have. Healthy hair starts from the inside. To see growth, you should have a healthy diet and stay hydrated. Some people use hair style as a form of personal expression. That is okay. Make sure that your parents/guardians approve of your hair style, along with your school or job.

PROBLEMS WITH HAIR GROWTH

HIRSUTISM

This occurs when there is an overgrowth of hair in the male pattern of distribution. The increase in hair may be related to an increase in a type of hormone. This hair may even grow on the face. There are many different causes of increased hair growth on the body. In order to find out why you have an overgrowth of hair, your health-care provider will want to know the age of onset, whether you have any other symptoms, and if you have used any medications.

HYPERTRICHOSIS

This is the name that is used when there is an increase in hair all over the body. This may happen suddenly or gradually. If you find that you have virilization (when a female develops masculine traits such as baldness, deepening of voice, and an increase in muscles) then you should see your health-care provider.

HAIR LOSS

Hair comes and goes. It has a cycle that includes growth, transition, and rest phases. For some, it may be normal to lose fifty to one hundred strands a day. Excessive hair loss can happen in adolescents for different reasons. The most common causes include stress, chronic health issues such as thyroid problems or polycystic ovary syndrome (see section on PCOS), or skin disorders. Check to make sure your diet is balanced as vitamin deficiency can also cause hair loss. Do not hesitate to bring it to your health-care provider's attention so they can investigate the cause or refer you to someone who can.

Absence of Hair (Alopecia)

This is when terminal hair does not develop where it would normally grow. This may be linked to genetics, but it may also be linked to illnesses such as diabetes, thyroid or kidney issues, and asthma, to name a few. This should be discussed with your health-care provider.

Summary Points

* The appearance of hair is one of the changes that characterize puberty.
* Methods can be used to control hair such as shaving, waxing, sugaring, depilatory creams, and trimming.
* You should be aware of the risks (bad things) and benefits (good things) about each method of hair control.
* Discuss the options with a parent or health-care provider when trying to determine which is the best for you.
* If you want to keep your hair, that is normal and okay.
* If you have problems with your hair growth such as too much hair or hair loss, bring this to the attention of your health-care provider.

CHAPTER 6

Adolescent Growth Spurt
and Bone Health

❧

Isaiah 58:11 (KJV)
And the Lord shall guide thee continually, and satisfy thy soul in drought, and make fat thy bones: and thou shalt be like a watered garden, and like a spring of water, whose waters fail not.

The adolescent growth spurt is the fast rate of growth and increase in weight that happens in your adolescent stage of life. It may start to happen before your adolescent years. Typically, your height will increase, your hips get wider, and you become more adult like. For example, my daughter was shorter than me last year. This year, she is almost as tall as I am. Your growth will continue until you are eighteen to nineteen years old. A small percentage of adolescents (up to ten percent) will not have a growth spurt or will have a small one.

During this time, most of the bones in your body will increase in length. Your bones are important because they have many functions. They carry your weight and support the body structurally. Bones allow us to move and protect organs such as the brain, heart, liver, lungs, and the female reproductive tract. Bones also act as a bank, storing minerals.

Bone mass and Age

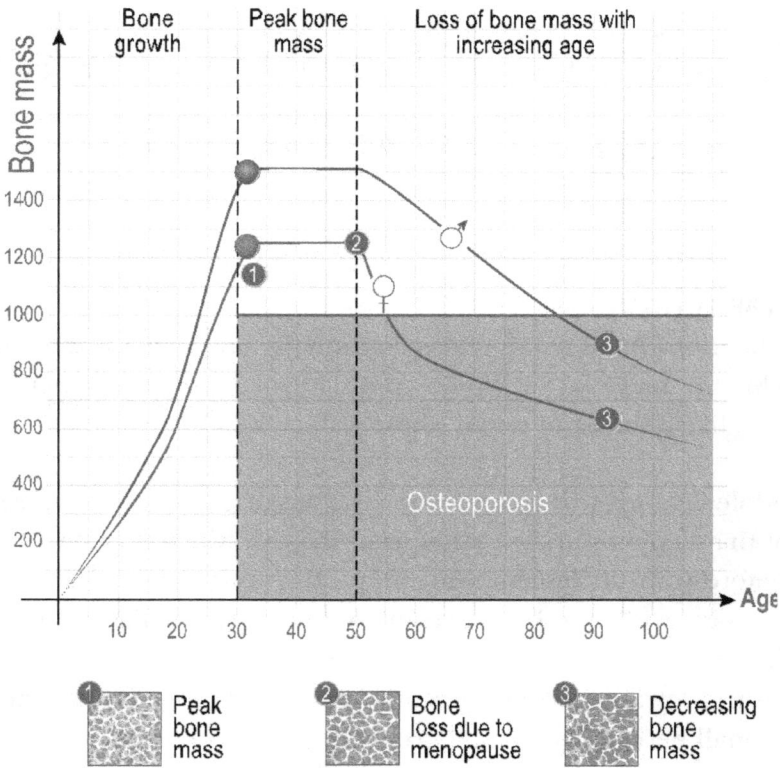

Figure 9. Bone mass and age

Peak bone mass (known as the bone bank) which you will draw upon for your entire adult life, is likely achieved by late adolescence, with the critical time for bone buildup happening much earlier. During adolescence, at least half of your peak bone mass is developed. You build up most of your bone bank before the age of twenty. Exercise can help bone to build up. Other things about you such as genetics (how you are made up), calcium/Vitamin D intake, your weight, medication intake, and general nutrition (what you eat) may also affect bone health. If you can increase your bone mass, this may decrease your risk of osteoporosis (thin bones) in adolescence and later in life.

Avoid activities that deplete the bone bank such as smoking and alcohol. Smoking encourages the production of cells that are responsible for resorption of the bone. It also decreases the formation of bone-producing cells. Smoking decreases blood supply to the bones, decreases absorption of calcium from your diet, and increases the rate of estrogen (an important hormone for bone health) breakdown and removal from the body. Alcohol can also affect bone health, as it causes different hormones in the body to increase, such as cortisol or parathyroid hormone, which decreases bone formation and removes calcium from the bone.

Healthy bones happen when you have proper nutrition (with adequate calcium and Vitamin D intake) and participate in regular physical activity (especially weight-bearing exercise). If you're an adolescent living with the average western diet and lifestyle, you may not be getting proper nutrition and exercise. It's important to make a deliberate effort to get enough calcium, a mineral that is crucial for bone development. Many sources of calcium and Vitamin D are available. Please see the list below.

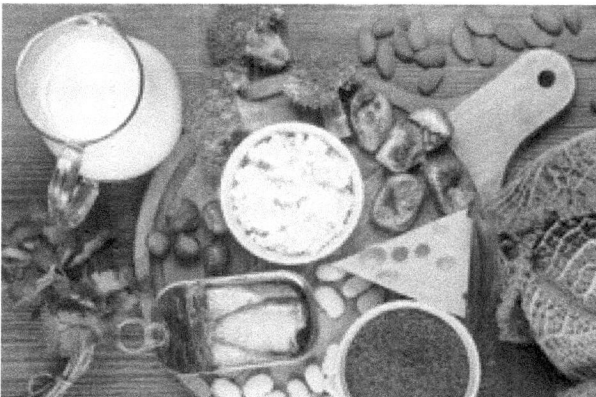

Figure 10. Sources of calcium

Calcium sources

* Dairy products, including milk, cheese, and yogurt
* Sesame, celery, and chia seeds
* Kale and collard greens
* Okra
* Broccoli and cabbage
* Almonds and figs
* Tofu
* Soybeans, edamame, beans, lentils, and pulse
* Some seafood including sardines, salmon, perch, rainbow trout, and shrimp
* Foods that are calcium fortified, such as orange juice, oatmeal, cereal, breads, and non-dairy milks

Vitamin D sources

* Sun exposure
* Fatty fish, such as tuna, mackerel, and salmon
* Foods fortified with Vitamin D, such as margarine, dairy products, orange juice, soy milk, and cereals
* Cheese
* Egg yolks
* Liver, beef, and cod liver oil

PARENTS AND GUARDIANS: HELP REDUCE THE RISK OF OSTEOPOROSIS

Strive to educate yourself and your family on the importance of dietary calcium and Vitamin D intake. Help create supportive environments in schools and in your community to encourage healthy diet and exercise habits. A bone-health screen that includes an assessment of calcium intake and determines whether there is a family history of adult osteoporosis (e.g., hip fracture, kyphosis) should be a routine part of adolescent health care.

ISSUES WITH BONE DEVELOPMENT AND HEALTH
SCOLIOSIS

Scoliosis is a sideways curvature of the spine. This curve may be C or S shaped and sometimes shows up after puberty. You may have symptoms such as back or leg pain, uneven hips or shoulders, difficulty standing up straight, or trouble walking. You may not have any symptoms. Your physician may notice scoliosis during your checkup. If this is the case, you will most likely be given a referral to see a specialist.

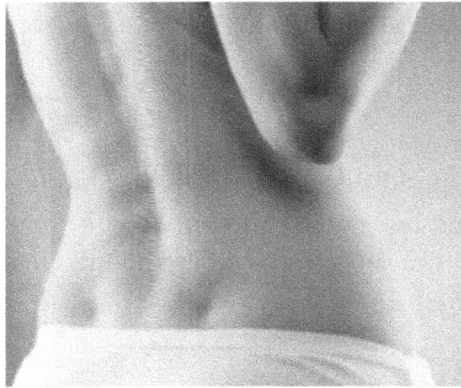

Figure 11. Scoliosis

OSTEOPOROSIS

Osteoporosis is a disease where the bones become thin and porous. This thinning of the bone usually does not happen in adolescence, but in rare cases it can occur, especially for those who have inherited a disease such as osteogenesis imperfecta. Those with irritable bowel disease, thyroid disease, kidney disease, anorexia nervosa, or who take high doses of medications that suppress the immune system (corticosteroids) are also at a higher risk for osteoporosis.

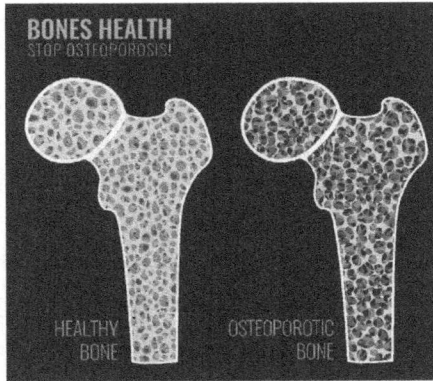

Figure 12. Normal bone compared to osteoporosis

Exercise

If you are in a competitive sport such as gymnastics, keep in mind that this can affect your hormones, and as a result, may affect your final height. Although exercise is important, competitive athletes may be at increased risk of fractures.

Bone Health Summary Points

* Bone is deposited and strengthened during adolescence, making it a key time for bone health.
* A balanced diet is important. Get enough Vitamin D and calcium.
* Exercise is important. Aim to get thirty to sixty minutes of moderate exercise daily.

* If you are on a diet, exercise a lot, or have a family history of osteoporosis, speak with your health-care provider.
* Avoid alcohol use.
* Avoid smoking, as this negatively affects bone health.
* Problems with bone, such as scoliosis or osteoporosis, can happen during adolescence.

CHAPTER 7

The First Period
—Is It Here Yet?

❧

WHAT IS MENSTRUATION?

The famed period, the monthly flow—that thing you look forward to
with either excitement or fear and the moment that can feel either cel-
ebrated or embarrassing. The average age for menstruation to begin is
twelve to thirteen years old. The age you start may be younger or older,
and is likely affected by your family history. Months before, you may
have noticed signs such as a change in body odor.

FIRST PERIOD

This is when the lining of the womb (uterus) breaks off and comes
out through the vagina. The amount of blood may be a little, a lot,
or somewhere in between. This event can carry different emotions.
It may catch you off guard if you have not thought about it or talked
about it yet. You may find it embarrassing, exciting, or you may think
it's no big deal.

No matter how you feel, it is a good idea to approach this major life
event with knowledge and prepare for it. I recommend talking to your
mother or sisters to find out the age they had their first period. Many
young ladies will have their period between ten and fourteen, about two
years after their breasts develop.

Your period usually comes once a month. The average time is every twenty-eight days, but for some it could come anywhere between every twenty-one and forty-five days. When it comes, it may last two to seven days.

Table 5
Average Menstruation Chart

	Normal	Not Normal
Duration	4–6 days	<2 days or >7 days
Volume	30 ml	>80 ml
Cycle Length	24–35 days	

Source: Treloar, et al. 1970. *International Journal of Fertility* 12:77.

Your period may come with or without cramps. You may not have any issues with your period or you may experience symptoms such as nausea, vomiting, or headaches. You may not be able to carry out your daily tasks. Normally, a period consists of a few tablespoons of blood. You may or may not have blood clots (a clump of blood that has changed from a liquid to a semisolid state). Bleeding, if heavy, may leave you tired, in pain, feeling down, and could affect your quality of life. If this is the case, you may have to take time off from school, extracurricular activities, or work. (Please see the section on issues with periods.)

WHY DOES A PERIOD HAPPEN?
In short, a period happens because of hormonal changes in your body. The longer answer is that a period involves the hypothalamus, pituitary, ovary, and uterus. The endometrium (lining of the womb) thickens as a result of the estrogen in your body and then changes when another hormone progesterone influences it. Then it breaks down when the hormones decrease. The period then stops because the blood clots and the uterus contracts. This process is controlled by local prostaglandins (substances that control different actions).

THE PHYSIOLOGY OF PUBERTY

Hormones change with the onset of puberty—the follicles produce hormones that are called sex hormones. This then affects the brain.

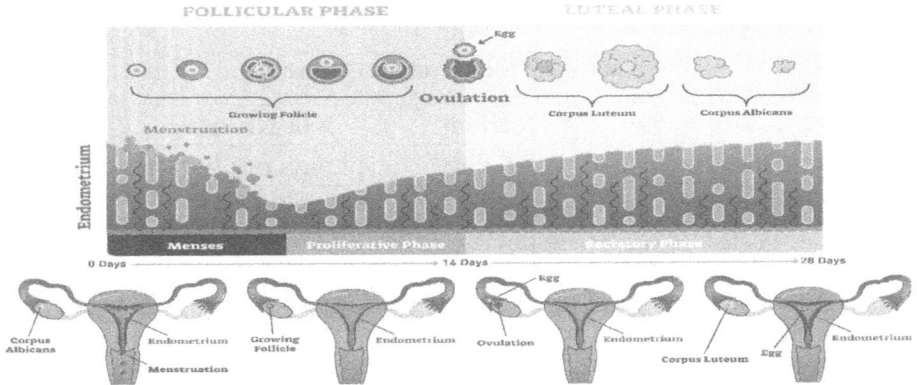

Figure 13. Female reproductive cycle

Changes are happening in different areas of the female system at the same time. Throughout the cycle, some hormones go up and some go down. This affects the cycle.

Your cycle is divided into parts. When talking about the ovaries, the terms used are *follicular phase, ovulatory phase*, and *luteal phase*. When talking about the womb, the terms used are *menses, proliferative phase*, and *secretory phase*.

THE HYPOTHALAMIC-PITUITARY AXIS

The hypothalamus, pituitary gland, and the ovaries have an intimate relationship. The actions of one impact the other. The changes in what is referred to as the hypothalamic-pituitary axis cause hormonal changes that affect the reproductive endocrine phases such as puberty and menstruation.

THE MENSTRUAL CYCLE

Throughout the month, your body has different processes going on in the organs that play a role in the female reproductive system, which conclude in a period. The pathways are complicated, and they are referred to as phases.

1. The follicular and luteal phases are based on the ovaries.
2. The proliferative and secretory phases are based on what is happening in the endometrium (lining) of the uterus.

ENDOMETRIUM

Throughout the month, under the influence of hormones, this lining of the womb is thickening and preparing to maintain a pregnancy. Once pregnancy does not take place and the cycle ends, much of the lining of the uterus (approximately two-thirds) leaves in the form of mostly blood and clots (period). Then the cycle starts over again.

OVULATION

I usually tell my patients that you are born with all the eggs that you will ever have. At puberty, you have roughly three hundred thousand to six hundred thousand follicles (oocytes). These have not matured. Maturity of the oocytes happens in stages, just like your development happens in stages. Once you go through puberty, a few are recruited each month for further development, as a result of the hormones (see hormone section). Eventually one (sometimes two) reach the final stages of development. These candidates are the ones that are released, which is called ovulation. The remainder then stop growing and disappear.

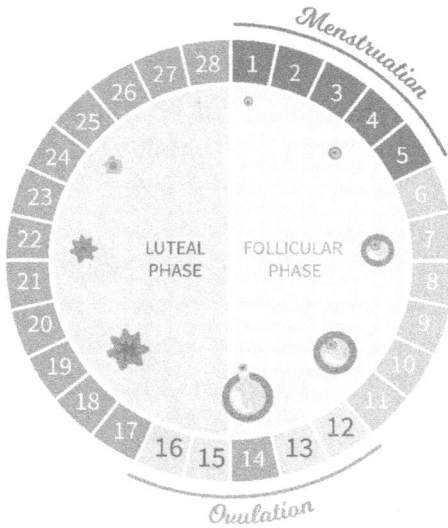

Figure 14. Human female menstrual cycle

DEALING WITH MENSTRUATION

If you do not have a severely painful period, no one has to know that you are on your period unless you want them to know. You can still participate in sports and go swimming on your period. A term for taking care of yourself during the period is *menstrual hygiene.*

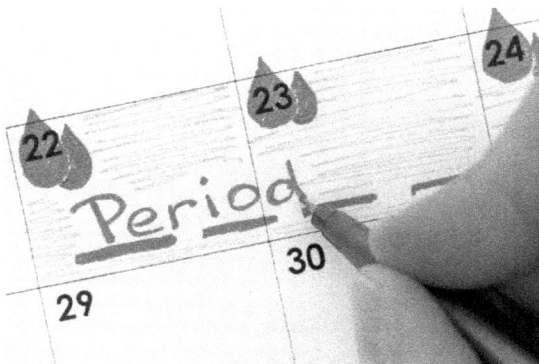

Figure 15. Marking a period on a calendar

Once your period becomes regular, you can use a calendar or a cell phone app to keep track of them. This makes it less likely that you'll be caught unprepared. Items that can be used during menstruation to catch the blood and keep you tidy include:

* Tampons
* A menstrual cup
* Panty liners
* Pads

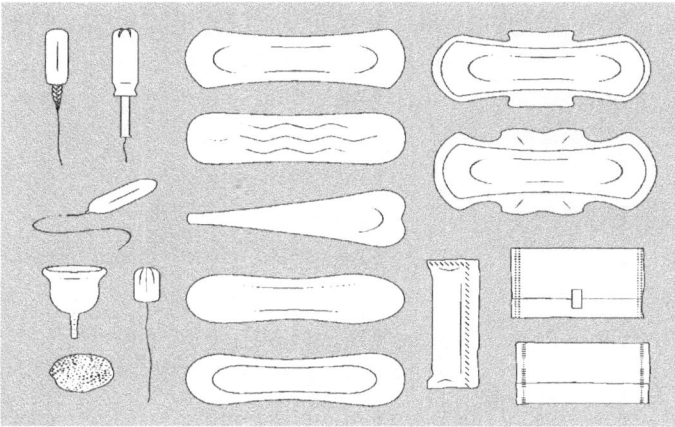

Figure 16. Options for keeping tidy during menses

Tampons have an applicator tube made of either cardboard or plastic that helps slide the tampon into place. Some tampons don't have an applicator tube and are just inserted with your finger. Tampons usually have a string at the end that enables you to remove them. You should change your tampon every four to eight hours or whenever it is uncomfortable. Tampons may be beneficial if you want to play sports or go swimming during your period.

A menstrual cup is a feminine hygiene product that is made of plastic or rubber. It is inserted into the vagina during your period. Its purpose is to prevent menstrual fluid (blood) from leaking onto one's clothes. The menstrual cup is emptied every four hours.

Pads are placed inside your underwear. They are designed to collect the menstrual flow. They can come in a variety of styles and sizes. They may have extra parts such as wings to help keep the pad in place and to capture any flow that may go over the side of the pad.

A panty liner is similar to a pad but is usually much thinner and designed to catch discharge or light spotting.

You may consider changing your pad, tampon, liner, or emptying your cup each time you urinate. Always keep some on you as sometimes the period comes a little before it is expected. Select products that are hypoallergenic as they are less irritating. Reusable and organic products are also available.

SUMMARY POINTS

* The period (menses) comes when the lining of the womb (endometrium) sheds.
* It happens because of hormonal changes in the body.
* It usually comes once a month but may be less frequent when the period first begins.
* Many products are available to help you remain tidy during your period such as tampons, menstrual cups, pads, and pantyliners.

CHAPTER 8

Period Issues

❦

AMENORRHEA—NO PERIOD HERE

Amenorrhea is when a person does not have a period. The most common reason for not having a period is that you are pregnant. But if you are not having sex and this happens, then this would not be the reason. There are a small percentage of ladies who have never had a period. You are considered to have amenorrhea if the period has not come by the age of fifteen or sixteen. If your breasts have not developed by twelve to thirteen, this is a reason to see your doctor.

Some causes of amenorrhea include:

* Constitutional delay in puberty
* Pregnancy
* Genetic causes
* Structural problems with the female reproductive system
* Hormonal issues
* Ovarian insufficiency
* Chronic health conditions such as obesity or eating disorders
* Pituitary mass

CONSTITUTIONAL DELAY OF PUBERTY

This happens when you reach puberty at an older age than the average age of sixteen to eighteen.

PREGNANCY

Pregnancy is the most common reason for the absence of a period. If you are not sexually active, then you are not able to become pregnant. But if you are sexually active, your health-care provider will give you a pregnancy test to check.

GENETIC CAUSES

Some genetic illnesses will cause your period not to come. For example, a female normally has two XX chromosomes. Chromosomes carry the information that make up who we are (genetics). But if your genetic makeup is different, you may not have a period. For example, an adolescent with Turner syndrome may only have one X chromosome. Other illnesses, such as androgen insensitivity syndrome or gonadal dysgenesis, can result in someone who looks female but may not have any internal reproductive organs or may have internal organs that are male. In these cases, the person will not have a menstrual cycle. If this condition is suspected, you will be referred to a reproductive endocrinologist who will advise you on the next steps in your care.

STRUCTURAL ISSUES WITH THE FEMALE GYNECOLOGIC SYSTEM

MULLERIAN ABNORMALITIES

This covers a range of conditions wherein a portion of the female reproductive system—such as the vagina, cervix, or uterus—is absent, smaller than normal, or duplicated. Imaging (e.g., an ultrasound) of the female parts may help your provider decide it this affects you. Some of these abnormalities have to be corrected with surgery. If your doctor believes that you have this, you will likely be referred to a pediatric gynecologist or a reproductive endocrinologist (a gynecologist who has done additional training to manage issues with the reproductive system).

IMPERFORATE HYMEN

The hymen is the tissue that covers the inside of the vagina. It may have different shapes and openings, which would only be seen and noted by your gynecologist. These openings allow the period to come through in someone who has never been sexually active (a virgin). In some cases, there are no openings in the hymen. This is called an imperforate hymen. This may cause your period not to come, as the tissue may block the flow of the period out of the vagina. If this is present, it will usually cause severe pain at the time of menses. If this is the case, surgery may be required to allow your period to come.

CERVICAL STENOSIS

When the neck of the womb opening is closed (stenotic) it can prevent the menses from leaving the womb. This could cause the absence of a period and pain. A gynecologist may have to do a procedure to open the area (dilate) so that the period can flow through.

HORMONAL ISSUES

Polycystic ovaries may start before or during adolescence. This condition can cause a change in the hormones and increase insulin resistance, which may delay menses. (See section on PCOS). You may also have some hirsutism (male-pattern hair growth). Some adolescents with this condition are overweight for their height.

PRIMARY OVARIAN INSUFFICIENCY

This is when the ovaries do not produce enough hormones to cause menses. Sometimes we are unable to figure out why this happens. In other cases, it may be caused by Fragile X syndrome, a problem with certain enzymes (which control how substances are broken down in the body), or a situation where the immune system produces substances that negatively affect the ovaries.

CHRONIC ILLNESSES, EATING DISORDERS, AND OBESITY
These conditions can make the hormones that normally cause a menstrual cycle be released in a way that stops it from happening.

PITUITARY MASS
A mass in the pituitary gland may cause an excess of a particular hormone that causes the period not to come.

SECONDARY AMENORRHEA
If the period comes and then goes away for more than six months, this is called secondary amenorrhea. The possible causes of this include Mullerian anomalies (a range of disorders where the anatomy may not be normal).

IRREGULAR PERIODS
When a period first starts, menstrual cycles (periods) may be irregular and range in length from twenty-one to forty-five days apart. You may skip periods in the second year after menstruation starts. This is a common concern but may be normal. Sometimes irregular periods can be caused by medications, exercise, or imbalances in the hormones. If do not have your period for several months in a row, you should see your health-care provider.

PREMENSTRUAL SYNDROME (PMS) OR PREMENSTRUAL DYSPHORIC DISORDER (PMDD)
Each month before a period starts, some ladies have symptoms. These symptoms start in the luteal phase of the cycle and resolve with the

menstrual cycle. In other words, the symptoms come four to five days before the period starts and stop by the fourth day of the period. The symptoms then remain absent until the next luteal phase. This is called premenstrual syndrome (PMS) or premenstrual dysphoric disorder (PMDD) (see section on mental health).

These symptoms can be emotional (affective), such as confusion, irritability, mood swings, outbursts, anxiety, depression, or withdrawal. The physical (somatic) symptoms may include weight gain, breast tenderness, stomach bloating, joint pain, headaches, nausea, or vomiting. They may affect your quality of life and ability to function in your daily activities.

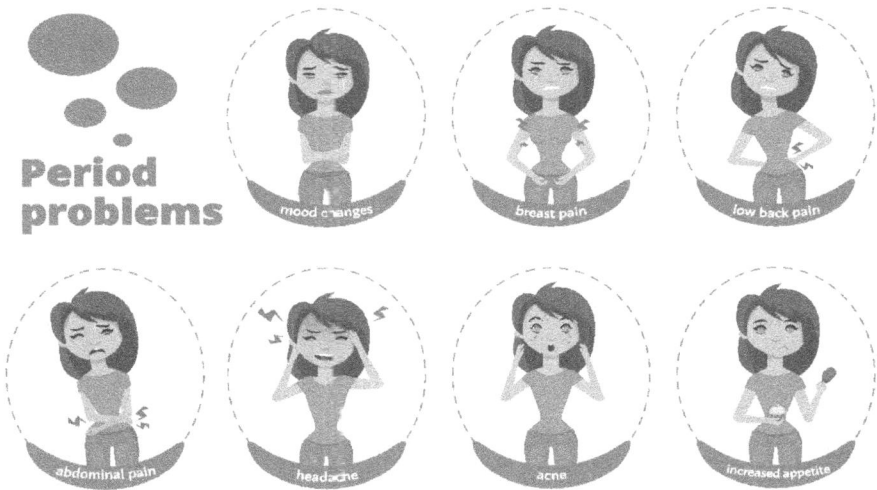

Figure 17. Symptoms that may come with a period

MENSTRUAL SYMPTOMS (MY PERIOD IS HERE—WHAT IS GOING ON!)

The hormone changes that happen which allow the period to come can affect other parts of the body too, including the nervous system, the skin, and the gut. You may find that you have stomach pain, headaches, skin breakouts, an increase in appetite, and sometimes an increase or decrease in the number of bowel movements (stools) you have. Some ladies find that their joints or muscles hurt. Sometimes you may feel bloated, tired, or have difficulty sleeping.

Quite frankly, there may be days when you do not want to be bothered. Make sure to discuss these symptoms with your provider, as we may have some simple solutions that can help. For example, pain medication may be available for the cramps and headaches. A heating pad or warm bath or shower may help with the abdominal and low back pain. The appetite changes and bloating may require changes to your diet and increased exercise.

If you have bad nausea with your periods, your health-care provider may recommend anti-nausea medicine. In some cases, birth control pills may be helpful. You should write down any symptoms that come with your period. Talk about them with your guardian and health care provider.

DYSMENORRHEA (MY PERIOD IS HERE, AND THIS HURTS!)

This is a crampy pain in the abdomen that starts with the beginning of the period and increases as the period continues. There are two types of dysmenorrhea—primary and secondary. Primary dysmenorrhea is when the pain is related to the hormones and changes with the menstrual cycle. Secondary dysmenorrhea occurs when there is something else that is causing the pain. Secondary dysmenorrhea can be caused by something in the pelvic region that is responsible for the pain, such as cysts (sacs filled with fluid that can be in or next to the ovary or fallopian tubes), congenital malformation, infection, fibroids, scar tissue in the pelvis, or endometriosis.

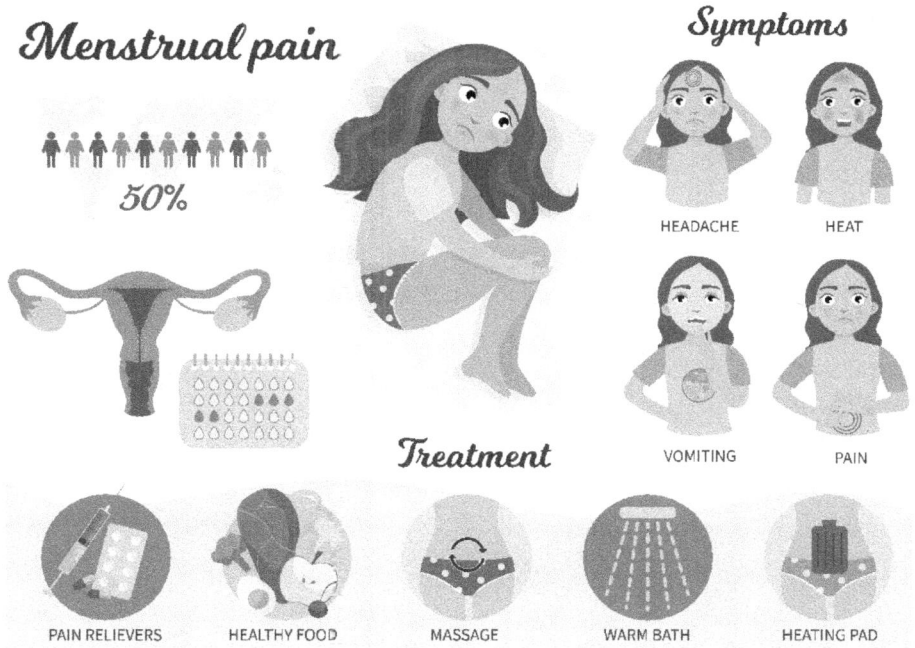

Figure 18. Ways to deal with menstrual pain and symptoms

ENDOMETRIOSIS

This occurs when the lining of the womb is located in other places besides the womb, so that when the lining is activated these other areas are activated as well. It is one of the most common reasons for pelvic pain in females, especially pain that does not improve with pain medication. This is the most common cause of secondary dysmenorrhea. Symptoms may worsen close to the time of menses.

These implants can be almost anywhere. In my experience, I have patients with it in the abdomen, in surgical scars, in the belly button, on the bladder, in the vagina, on the ovaries, outside of the uterus, and in the space behind and lateral to the womb. Endometriosis may cause other issues aside from pain with the menstrual cycle, including pain with bowel movements, stomach pain, pain with sex, and difficulties getting pregnant. It can be extremely challenging to diagnose and to treat. Most adolescents will have a normal exam when reviewed with their presenting symptoms.

Sometimes, an ultrasound, magnetic resonance imaging (MRI, a special test used to see tissues), and a surgical procedure may assist in the diagnosis. There are medications that can be used to suppress the hormones and possibly improve symptoms. If the medications are not helpful, diagnostic laparoscopy (keyhole surgery) may confirm the diagnosis of endometriosis. This is when we look into the abdomen to determine whether we can see any of the endometrial tissue. Removing that tissue may improve symptoms in a person with endometriosis. We should also remember that some ladies have endometriosis and have no symptoms.

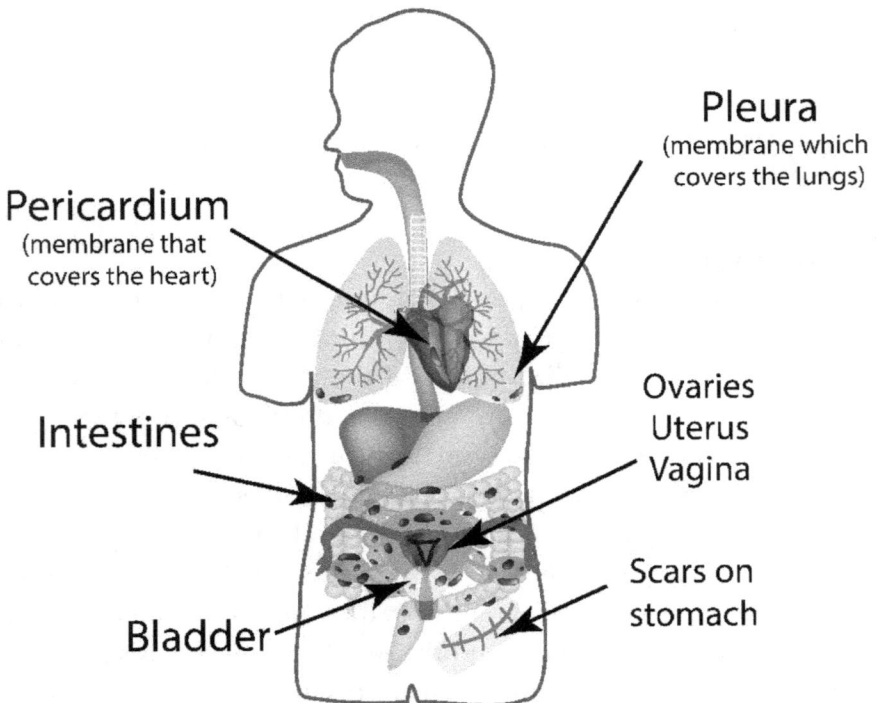

Figure 19. Some Sites of Endometriosis

FIBROIDS

These are non-cancerous growth that are caused by hormones—especially estrogen. Fibroids are uncommon in adolescence, but they have been reported. They may cause abnormal bleeding or pain. Fibroids have different names depending on where they are located in relation to the uterus.

Types of uterine fibroids

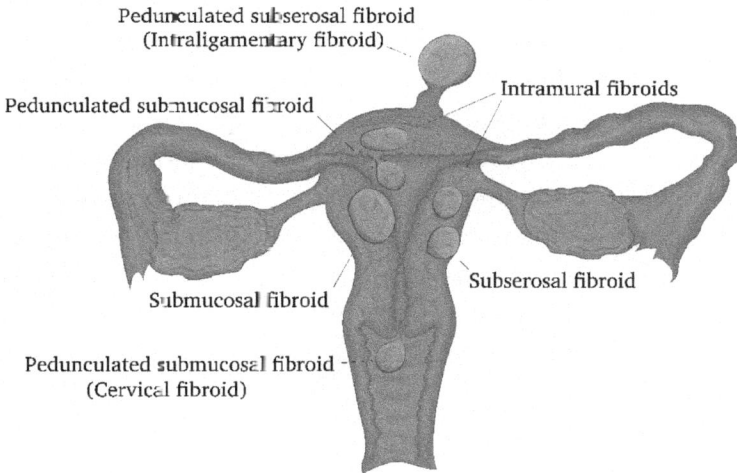

Pedunculated subserosal fibroid
(Intraligamentary fibroid)

Pedunculated submucosal fibroid

Intramural fibroids

Submucosal fibroid

Subserosal fibroid

Pedunculated submucosal fibroid
(Cervical fibroid)

Figure 20. Types of uterine fibroids

TUBERCULOSIS

This infection is caused by Mycobacterium tuberculosis. Genital tuberculosis usually occurs when a lung tuberculosis infection has spread to other parts of the body. Genital tuberculosis affects the female genital organs—the ovaries, fallopian tubes, vagina, cervix, and lymph nodes. This too can be a cause of pelvic pain or infertility in the future. You have to keep this in mind if you have been exposed to someone who has tuberculosis. If your health-care provider suspects tuberculosis, they would do a simple skin test and then additional tests as needed.

Heavy or Prolonged Menses (My Period Will *Not* Stop!)

Some adolescents have difficulty with their menses. Their period may go on for longer than normal (eight days) or they may bleed more than normal. This can cause your red blood cell count to drop. As a result, you may feel tired or worn down. You may also have to stop activities that you would normally do.

A heavy cycle or a cycle that lasts longer than normal in your age group may be related to hormonal changes and may be caused by anovulatory cycles. These are periods where you may not release an egg (ovulate). Heavy cycles in your age group may also be caused by bleeding disorders. Heavy periods can be managed by hormonal means, such as the birth control pill or progesterone-type medication, depending on what your health-care provider thinks is causing the bleeding.

Your health-care provider may check your complete blood count (CBC), thyroid function, and Von Willebrand factor. Sometimes, if your bleeding is heavy or prolonged, you may need to take iron supplements to try to keep your blood count up and avoid anemia. If the problem is related to your thyroid gland, you may need medication. If it is related to the way that your blood clots, you may need medication to help with that.

Summary Points

* If your period does not come by age fifteen or sixteen you should bring it to the attention of your health-care provider.
* You may not have a period because of structural issues.
* If you have painful periods, let a guardian and health-care provider know.
* If you have heavy periods or your period lasts for longer than a week, let your guardian and health-care provider know.

CHAPTER 9

Vulvar Issues in Adolescence

❧

THE VULVAR AREA

The lips of the vagina may have issues from time to time. For example, they may become irritated or stick together. Conditions frequently seen include vulvovaginitis, vulvar irritation from hygiene products, or chronic conditions of the vulva.

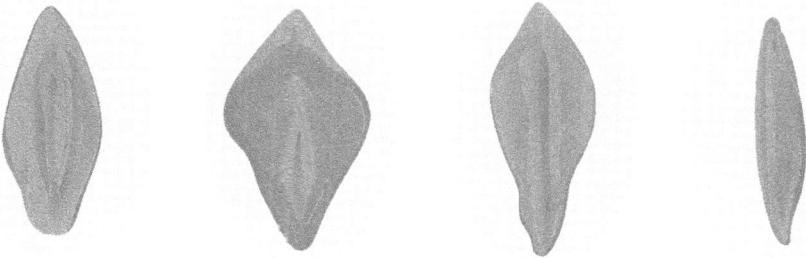

Figure 21. Some different vulvar shapes

LABIAL ADHESIONS

This occurs when the lips of the vagina are stuck together. This usually affects prepubertal patients (those who haven't started puberty) as opposed to pubertal (those who have reached puberty) patients. Your doctor may provide some medication to keep the lips from sticking to one another.

Vulvovaginitis

At puberty the environment in the vagina changes. It becomes acidic to help protect you from vaginal irritations. We group these irritations under the term vulvovaginitis. They often cause a vaginal discharge and or itching. There may be a lot or a little discharge and it may be white, yellow, or grey in color and creamy or lumpy.

Vulvovaginitis might make the area feel painful, swollen, irritated, or itchy. It may even burn when you urinate. Take note of when your symptoms started, the color of any discharge, whether there is itching, or if you have been on any medication recently. Causes of the discharge may include:

* Bacterial infections
* Fungal infections
* Parasitic infections
* Allergic vaginitis/bubble bath vaginitis
* Urethral prolapse
* Lichen sclerosus
* Poor hygiene
* Sexual abuse

Bacterial Infections

There are many different types of bacteria on the skin. When certain bacteria increase too much and cause an imbalance, they may cause discharge and irritation. Sometimes, we do a swab (culture) of the area to determine which bacteria is causing the problem. If we are able to figure out which bacteria is the culprit, we call it a specific vaginitis. Sometimes we are not able to figure out exactly which bacteria is causing the problem. We call this a non-specific vaginitis. An infection elsewhere in the body can also be passed to the vulva (if you have a stomach infection that causes diarrhea, for example). The same bacteria that caused the bacteria can get into the vagina and cause discharge.

FUNGAL INFECTIONS

Yeast (candida) infections are not common in adolescents but they can happen. Sometimes when they occur often (recurrent) that can be a sign of something more serious such as diabetes or a weakened immune system.

PARASITES

Worm infections are common. They may live in the colon and travel out at night. If they get into the vagina this may cause discharge and itching.

ALLERGIC CONTACT DERMATITIS

We often like to use bath products that smell nice or are in nice packaging. As a young lady, bubble baths and bath bombs were some of my favorite gifts to give and receive. Unfortunately, products such as soaps, bath wash, and detergents can cause irritation in the vagina. The area may become itchy, red, or swollen. You may or may not have discharge. To address this problem, you have to stop using the agent causing the problem. You can also do sitz baths (a warm shallow bath) with oatmeal or baking soda to help relieve the irritation. See your doctor as you may need additional treatment to soothe the inflammation.

URETHRAL PROLAPSE

If the urethra's two muscle layers separate, the mucosa can stick out through the opening of the urethra. The mucosa may become swollen and red/purple. It may even bleed and cause vaginal discharge. This may cause you to be unable to pee (urinary retention) or have pain when you pee. This is rare in adolescents, but it can happen.

LICHEN SCLEROSUS

This is a problem where there is an abnormal thickening in the vulva area. This may cause the area to be itchy and have a shiny whitish color. This should be reviewed with your gynecologist.

POOR HYGIENE

Poor hygiene can allow different types of bacteria to build up which will then need to be treated with antibiotics and with careful attention to keeping the vulva clean. It is best to use a mild soap and water to cleanse the vulva and ensure that you wipe the creases between the labia minora and labia majora.

SEXUAL ABUSE

Sexual abuse can cause vaginal discharge, bruising, or vaginal spotting. This can be difficult to consider as an adolescent or parent, but it happens.

BARTHOLIN'S DUCT CYST/ABSCESS

This is a gland in the vagina that can become swollen. If you have this, your doctor may decide to monitor it. Sometimes bacteria can get into it and cause pain. If this is the case, your doctor may decide to treat and remove the infection. Treatment may involve antibiotics and draining the area (incision and drainage). If you have a Bartholin's abscess and you've been sexually active, your doctor may suggest checking for other-infections, such as gonorrhea and chlamydia.

ENDOMETRIOSIS

Tissue that normally lines the womb may be found in any other location, including the vulva and vagina. These spots may look purple and can cause bleeding or spotting around the time of your period.

LIPOMA

A lipoma is a fatty, non-cancerous, soft tissue tumor that can be found anywhere in the body. Lipomas have been reported in adolescents in the vulva. The exact cause is not known. They can be removed surgically.

LABIAL HYPERTROPHY

If one or both of the lips of the vagina are increased in size, it can cause infection or irritation. If you have this but it is not causing you any issues, your health-care provider may just monitor it. However, if it is causing problems, your health-care provider may recommend that you see a specialist to change the size of the area.

HEMANGIOMA (HAMARTOMA)

These strawberry-colored lesions may be flat or raised. They usually appear during childhood and get smaller with time or possibly disappear. This condition is rare in your age group.

SCABIES AND CRAB LICE

The skin on the vulva is also prone to infection by parasites. The two most common culprits are scabies and crab lice. These are transmitted by close contact from objects such as towels or bedding or through sexual contact. They both cause itching and may result in bumps in the area. The treatment of both involves a medicine that kills the parasite and destroys its eggs. It is recommended that, if diagnosed, all persons who have been in close contact with the affected person also be treated.

VULVAR ULCERS

Vulvar ulcers affect the top layer of skin (epidermis) and the layer underneath (dermis). They are sores that can have a regular or irregular border, may appear to be a different color from your normal skin color, may be single, many, sunken, heaped up, and recurrent.

Vulvar ulcers can be caused by bacteria or viruses, including herpes, human papillomavirus, syphilis, Staphylococcus, and chlamydia. Painful ulcers in young ladies who have never been sexually active may be a result of infection of the vulva with viruses such as cytomegalovirus, Epstein-Barr virus, or the flu (Influenza A). Non-infectious ulcers can also be caused by medications. Ulcers can also be a sign of other illnesses that may affect the entire body, such as Crohn's disease, Behcet's syndrome, or trauma. If you have an ulcer, bring it to the attention of your health-care provider. A biopsy may be required to help determine its cause.

NEUROFIBROMATOSIS

This is a hereditary disorder of the nervous system that causes problems with balance and hearing. There are two different types. It usually causes growths that may look like nodules. These lesions may also appear on the vulva.

PIGMENTED AREAS (MELANOCYTES, MOLE, AND NEVI)

You may have areas that appear brown or purple. These can be anywhere on the vulva. They are usually nothing to be concerned about but you should let a health-care provider review and assess them to make sure they are not caused by a concerning condition such as melanoma (a type of cancer).

Summary Points

* You can have problems with the lips of the vagina (vulva).
* If you have problems when you use products such as soaps, body washes, or bubble baths, stop using them.
* If you have an abnormal discharge, bring it to the attention of your health-care provider.
* If you have an ulcer, bring it to the attention of your health-care provider.
* If you have nodules or a colored area, notify your health-care provider so they can explain what it is to you.

CHAPTER 10

Issues with the Ovaries in Adolescence

OVARIAN CYSTS

Ovarian cysts are fluid-filled sacs found in the ovaries. Non-cancerous cysts can be divided into functional and non -functional cysts. Functional cysts are a result of the normal process that happens in the ovaries (ovulation). These are corpus luteum cysts or follicular cysts. Non-functional cysts are not a part of the normal process in the ovaries. A cyst that has endometrial tissue is an endometrioma. One that has bleeding in it, a hemorrhagic cyst. If a cyst has tissue in it that is found in other parts of the body such as hair, teeth or bone it is called a teratoma (dermoid). A cyst that forms next to the ovary, a paraovarian cyst.

OVARIAN CYSTS

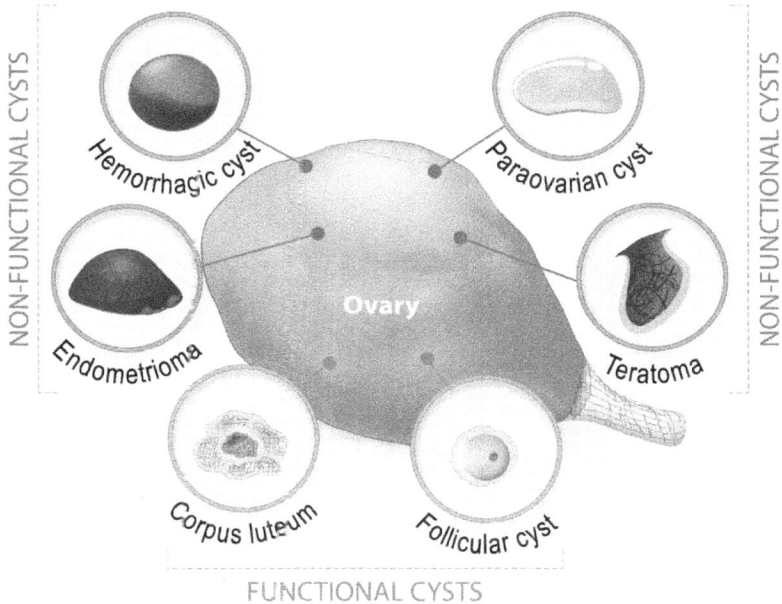

Figure 22. Types of non-cancerous ovarian cysts

These may not cause any symptoms, or sometimes they may break open and release the fluid or twist, causing pain in the stomach or the side. If the cyst is increasing in size or causing pain, your doctor may recommend surgery to remove it. The good news is that many cysts in your age group do not increase in size and go away with time. You may be placed on hormonal medication such as oral contraceptive pills to decrease the chance that you will form additional cysts.

POLYCYSTIC OVARY SYNDROME

Polycystic ovary syndrome (PCOS) is an endocrine disorder that is not fully understood but affects several different glands and organs, including the pituitary gland, ovaries, adrenal glands, and fat cells. As a result, you may have abnormal cycles and signs of excess androgens such as hirsutism. The ovaries may not release a follicle each month. In fact, they may not fully development. Sometimes, this can be seen on pelvic ultrasound (an exam that gives images to check the structures). PCOS is found in four out of one hundred adolescents. This diagnosis is usually made at least two years after the start of your period. It may be the reason for the late start of your period.

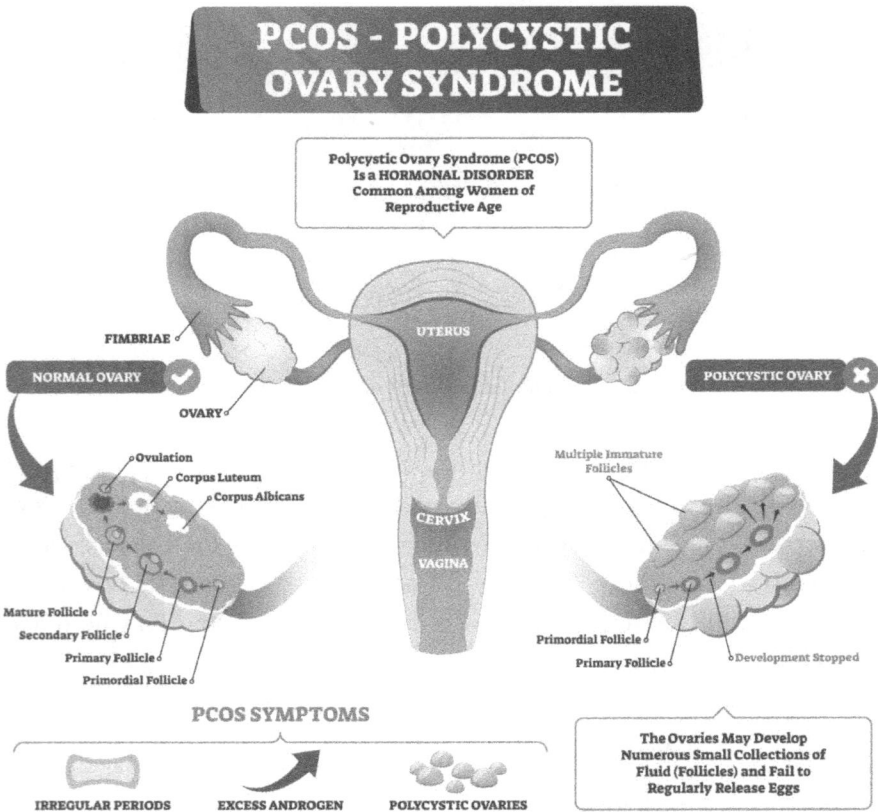

Figure 23. Comparison of ovary with PCOS compared to a normal ovary

PCOS can cause problems in adulthood with weight and the ability to get pregnant. It can also cause problems in adolescence such as acne, increased body hair, irregular periods, fatigue, cysts in the ovaries, or difficulty with losing weight.

PCOS SYMPTOMS

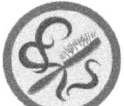
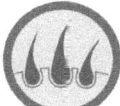
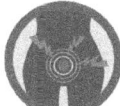

HAIR LOSS　　**HIRSUTISM**　　**PELVIC PAIN**

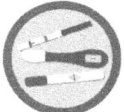
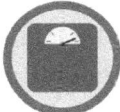
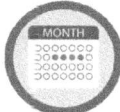

INFERTILITY　　**OVERWEIGHT**　　**IRREGULAR PERIODS**

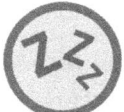
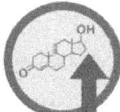
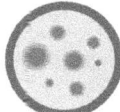

FATIGUE　　**HIGH TESTOSTERONE LEVELS**　　**ACNE**

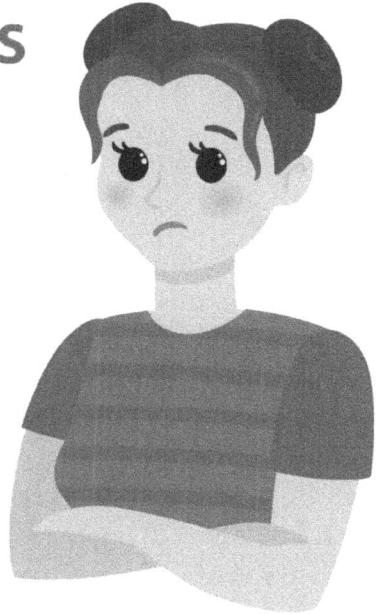

Figure 24. Symptoms of polycystic ovaries

Table 6

Effects of Polycystic Ovary Syndrome		
Prepubertal	Adolescence	Reproductive Years
Early puberty	Irregular menstrual cycles Hirsutism Hair Loss Fatigue Acne Obesity Insulin resistance Glucose intolerance Decrease in quality of life Pelvic Pain	Type II Diabetes Mellitus Infertility Hypertension Low Sex Drive Pelvic Pain

Some of the ways that we evaluate for this include taking a clinical history or doing an exam. Your provider may also recommend an ultrasound scan of the pelvis. Some ways that this issue is managed include lifestyle changes such as diet and exercise. Medications may also be recommended to assist with the symptoms (e.g., to treat menstrual irregularities).

PELVIC PAIN

Chronic pelvic pain is when a person experiences pelvic pain for at least three to six months. This happens in three out of ten ladies. It can cause frustration, suffering, absence from school, or inability to participate in social activities. Sometimes the pain is caused by problems with other parts of the body, such as the appendix, stomach, intestines, colon, or bladder.

If the pain is related to the female organs, it is separated into two groups: secondary dysmenorrhea (pain caused by something structural) or primary dysmenorrhea (pain caused by something that is nonstructural). The most common cause of recurrent pain is menstruation. Chronic pelvic pain is a common cause of visits to the gynecologist.

Primary dysmenorrhea is common, and many teenagers experience it. It is thought to be related to the hormones (prostaglandins) that cause the uterus to contract (squeeze). Medicine that decreases these hormone levels and decreases inflammation are used as treatment. You are also encouraged to have a healthy diet including lots of vitamin-rich vegetables and to reduce your refined sugar intake.

MITTELSCHMERZ

If you have pain in the lower part of your abdomen around midcycle, when your body releases an egg (ovulation), this could be mittelschmerz. Sometimes this pain is strong; but, it does not last long. The pain may be a result of irritation from the fluid released by the ruptured follicle. It may happen fourteen days before your period comes again.

This pain may be:

* Crampy in nature
* Felt on one side
* Dull or sharp in intensity
* Sudden in onset

Often a heating pad and some pain relievers help. The pain is usually not bad, but if it is, then you should see your doctor to review ways of dealing with it.

TORSION

Torsion is when an organ twists or rotates, usually on itself. In the female system, it can happen to the fallopian tubes or ovaries. If this is not diagnosed and treated, blood flow to the organ can decrease and the organ may stop functioning. This may cause pain that is severe. You may also have nausea and vomiting. The risk factors for torsion include having had a torsion before, having ovarian cysts, having longer than normal attachments (ligaments) that suspend the ovaries, or having an ovary that is increased in size. Torsion is a gynecologic emergency. If you think you have this issue, seek help immediately.

SUMMARY POINTS

* Adolescents can have problems with the ovaries, including cysts, endometriosis, and twisting of the ovaries.
* If you have polycystic ovarian syndrome, your cycles may be irregular. PCOS may have effects on your body later in life.

* Pelvic pain is common in adolescence and can have different causes. If you are having pain in the pelvic area it is important to see your health-care provider to find out why you are having the pain and how to manage it.
* If you have a torsion, it is an emergency.

CHAPTER 11

Screening in Adolescents

❧

SCREENING IS WHEN WE, AS health-care providers, try to prevent a disease. We estimate your chance of having a disease and look for any evidence of that disease process. We use a combination of things like talking to you, examining you, and conducting lab tests and studies to help you. In other words, we try to identify possible problem areas before they become a problem and make changes so that they do not become a problem.

Some of the things that you may be screened for include high blood pressure, diabetes, high cholesterol, sexually transmitted infections (STIs), eating disorders, depression, problems at school, emotional or sexual abuse, and use of tobacco, alcohol, or other substances.

PAP TEST

This is a screening test for cervical cancer, which is caused by high risk HPV (see chapter 11). This test is usually recommended at age twenty-one if you are having or have had sex. If you are not sexually active, you can put off having this test. Please talk about this with your health-care provider. You can breathe easy—your risk of cervical cancer is decreased with the HPV vaccine.

ABUSE

Abuse is when you are mistreated. Abuse can be physical, sexual, emotional, or can come from neglect. Abuse may be common in the adolescent years but may not be noticed. You may be hurt by those who are close to you, such as a person you are dating. This abuse can increase your chance of depression (feeling down for a prolonged period of time). Questions that you can ask yourself to determine whether you are a victim of abuse include the following:

* Has anyone touched you in a way that you do not want?
* Has anyone ever tried to have sex with you when you did not want them to?
* Has anyone ever hit or physically harmed you?
* Does anyone you interact with regularly make you feel scared—especially a family member or significant other?
* Has anyone tried to make you do something that you were not comfortable with?

Physical abuse may leave visible signs such as bruising and blemishes. Sexual abuse may cause vaginal discharge from sexual and/or non-sexual infections. It can also result in a pregnancy. Sexual abuse may negatively impact your sexual health, resulting in you taking unhealthy risks or not wanting to be sexually active in the future. In no shape or form is abuse normal—it is wrong. Think of your most favorite item and the care and attention you pay to it. Then think about how much more care and attention should be paid to you, who is so precious!

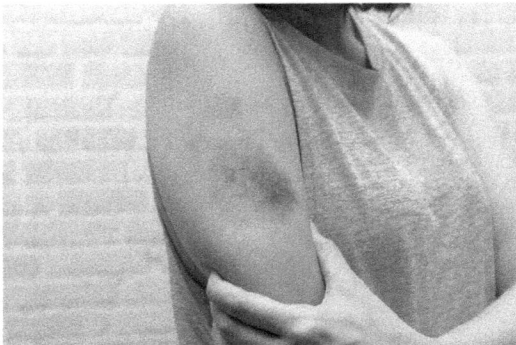

Figure 25. Bruises from physical abuse

Psalm 139:13-14 (KJV)
For thou hast possessed my reins: thou hast covered me in my mother's womb.

I will praise thee: for I am fearfully and wonderfully made: marvelous are thy works; and that my soul knoweth right well.

BULLYING

Bullying is when someone tries to harm or humiliate you. Most bullying goes unreported. Bullying can make you feel helpless. You may think that you can handle it by yourself or you may be afraid of the bully's response if you report it. Many bullying incidents happen in front of bystanders and many incidents stop when bystanders speak up.

Do you feel safe in school? If not, it is important to try to figure out why. What happens to you now may have a large impact on your future. Adolescence is hard. But when people make you feel uncomfortable or unhappy because of what they say or do, it can make things tougher.

Cyberbullying is when people use the Internet to harass you on a social media site or through digital devices like your cell phone. This may involve threats, sexual remarks, or hate words. The purpose of this is to make you feel bad. Sometimes, you can tell you are being bullied if you get a mean tweet or text. Sometimes someone may use photos, videos, or personal information to embarrass or hurt you. The person who is receiving this treatment may feel scared, frustrated, angry, or depressed.

Sometimes people may use the Internet as a way to get another person to react or for their own personal amusement. It can be difficult to tell someone that you are being bullied, but it is common. It is important to let someone whom you trust know what is happening. If left unresolved, being bullied can cause you problems in the future and affect the way that you feel about yourself. People who are bullied have an increased chance of feeling like hurting themselves.

To Prevent Bullying

* **Pay attention to the signs of bullying.**
* **Let your parents, teachers, and counsellors know if it is happening to you or another student.**
* **Talk about it.**
* **Check to see what policies your school has to prevent bullying and to penalize bullies.**

Sexual Harassment

When a person's comments concern your body, or if a person tries to touch you, this is called sexual harassment. The harasser may be someone that you know or may be a stranger. Whoever it is, what they are doing is wrong! Trust how you feel. If a person (or what they say) makes you feel uncomfortable or scared—pay attention. Whether the person is someone you know or not, it should stop. Let an adult you trust know what is happening.

Alcohol

As an adolescent, you are more at risk for the negative effects of alcohol on your brain. Research indicates that the brain continues to develop into your twenties. Since your brain is not yet fully developed, you may not anticipate the consequences of alcohol and may not be able to accurately evaluate the risk and reward. Drinking can lead to impaired judgement and decision making. For example, you may be more likely to engage in high risk behaviors such as sexual activity or drug use while intoxicated. You may also increase your risk of injury to yourself and others.

Smoking

Tobacco comes in many forms, such as cigarettes, cigars, bidis, chewable tobacco, electronic cigarettes, and hookah. You may see your peers, friends, or family members smoking. Smoking as an adolescent can affect your lungs and blood vessels, leading to heart disease. It may also affect your growth and cause cancer. Not to mention, the smoke tends to make your hair, skin, and clothes stink.

Vaping is when an e-cigarette or vape pen is used to make a vapor that can be inhaled.

Vaping with nicotine and other substances may initially increase your alertness and attention but in the long term can interfere with your lungs, cause changes in the brain, be addictive, and even lead to death.

DRUGS

There are different types of drugs such as weed, heroin, cocaine, meth-amphetamines, prescription pain medications, etc. The list goes on as new versions of old drugs and various new drugs are made. We may not understand the long- and short-term effects of all the drugs, but we know that they have an impact on the brain and the way it works. The drugs may make the user feel good for a short time, with a long-term price of destruction with continued use. They may negatively affect your relationship with yourself and others. I encourage you to "Just Say No to Drugs and Say Yes to Life."

PORNOGRAPHY (PORN)

Pornography includes television programs, magazines, media, and/or books (written or digital material) that contain explicit depictions of sexual activity.

When adolescents are exposed to porn, it changes their attitude to sex and may decrease their self-esteem when it comes to sex. It is reported to affect the brain in a similar way to drugs and alcohol. Although porn is designed to increase sexual excitement, it may also increase feelings of loneliness, depression, and shame.

SUMMARY

* Pay attention to any illnesses that are in the family.
* Ask your health-care provider for screening that is recommended for your age group.
* If you are a bully or participating in cyber harassment—*stop!*
* If you are being bullied or suspect you are a victim of any type of abuse, let your parent, guardian, or an adult you trust know what is happening. Tell a school counselor or someone in authority at the school.
* Choices are key in life. Some choices may affect your life for the long term.
* Avoid smoking and vaping.
* Avoid alcohol.
* Avoid abuse of prescription medications including pain killers.
* Be careful what you allow yourself to be exposed to, especially by the Internet and with peers.

1 Corinthians 15:33 (NIV)
Do not be misled: "Bad company corrupts good character."

1 Corinthians 13:11 (KJV)
When I was a child, I spake as a child, I understood as a child, I thought as a child: but when I became a man, I put away childish things.

CHAPTER 12

Let's Talk about Sex

❦

Matthew 6:26 (NIV)
Look at the birds of the air; they do not sow or reap or store away in barns, and yet your heavenly Father feeds them. Are you not much more valuable than they?

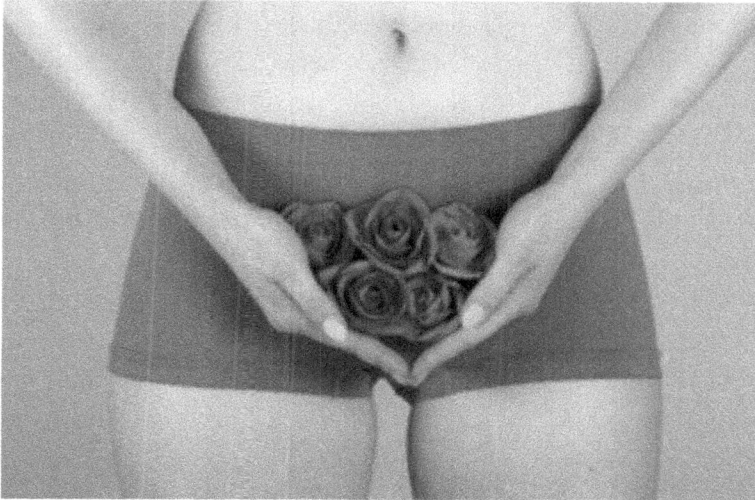

No one reaches mature adulthood without first going through adolescence and young adulthood. If you have questions about sex, speak with your parents, a counselor, and your health-care provider. As a health-care provider, I always encourage you to communicate with your parent or guardian. There is a good chance that an adult you know has been through similar experiences and has felt what you are feeling. It is important for you to know that as health-care providers, we are committed to keeping you in the very best of health. We have taken an oath to "Do no harm." With that in mind, we are willing to discuss topics that are important to your overall well-being.

Remember, you are special! You are valuable! Although you and your friends may know a lot, your friends do not know everything, and neither do you. Sex is important. It is the action that is responsible for the majority of the population. It plays a role in many healthy adult relationships. Like relationships, it can be complicated and should be approached with a mature outlook and attitude.

Sex is like a gun. If placed in the wrong hands, it can cause damage beyond your imagination. Although sex is beautiful, it can also cause irreparable damage when entered into without wisdom and without understanding the results of being sexually active.

Sex is defined as sexual contact between individuals which can involve penetration (one body part going into another, known as penetrative intercourse) or one part getting close to another part (known as non-penetrative or outer course). Sex can be broken down into different types, depending on which body parts are involved, including:

* Vaginal
* Oral
* Anal
* Digital

Both penetrative and non-penetrative sex have possible risks, including pregnancy and sexually transmitted infections (STIs). The only way to completely protect yourself from pregnancy or STI risk is to abstain from all sexual activities.

SEXUALLY TRANSMITTED INFECTIONS (STIs)/SEXUALLY TRANSMITTED DISEASES (STDs)

STIs and STDs (both mean the same thing) are infections that you are exposed to through sexual contact. They are passed from one person to another. STIs are no joke. If you are sexually active, whether its vaginal, anal, oral, or using fingers, you are at risk of picking up an STI. Some of these infections are treatable and some are lifelong.

STIs can be caused by bacteria, viruses, or fungus. Some STIs have symptoms and some do not. Even if you have an STI with no signs or symptoms, if you do not get treated, it may interfere with your life later. It could even affect your lifespan, the lifespan of someone you care about, and your ability to have children in the future. It could cost you money and time dealing with the complications. STIs tend to hang together. If you have one, it increases your chance of getting other STIs.

The most common types of STIs are:

* Gonorrhea
* Chlamydia
* Syphilis
* Trichomoniasis
* HSV (Herpes)
* HIV/AIDS (Human Immunodeficiency Virus, Acquired Immune Deficiency Syndrome)
* PID (Pelvic Inflammatory Disease)
* HPV (Human Papillomavirus)
* Zika
* HEPATITIS B AND HEPATITIS C

GONORRHEA

The bacterium *Neisseria gonorrhoeae* can grow and multiply quickly in the right environment, which happens to be your reproductive tract. This infection may not have symptoms, but some may have symptoms such as vaginal discharge, bleeding in between periods, pain in the stomach, or an increase in frequency of urination (pee). The sooner you get treated, the better, as it can cause long-term irreversible harm to your reproductive parts. It can also affect the mouth, throat, eyes, and bottom (rectum). If you have gonorrhea, it changes your cells in a way that makes it easier to get HIV. Gonorrhea is treated with antibiotics.

CHLAMYDIA

This is caused by a bacterium called *Chlamydia trachomatis.* You can get this infection in the cervix, the rectum, or the throat. Some people may not have symptoms, but others can have pain in the abdomen, fever, and discharge from the vagina. If left untreated, it could affect your ability to get pregnant or cause an eye or lung infection. However, once chlamydia is diagnosed, it is easily treatable with antibiotics.

SYPHILIS

This is an STI that is caused by a bacterium called *Treponema pallidum.* It is treated with penicillin. Catching it and treating it early can prevent long-term damage to the heart, brain, and liver. Syphilis has different stages: primary, secondary, and tertiary. A person may have no symptoms or may have painful bumps (sores).

TRICHOMONIASIS

Trichomoniasis is caused by the protozoan-*Trichomonas vaginalis.* A person with Trichomoniasis may have no symptoms or may have a colored vaginal discharge, vaginal burning, redness, itching, or an increased need to urinate. Trichomoniasis is treatable with antibiotics.

HERPES SIMPLEX VIRUS (HSV)

There are two types of HSV: Type I and Type 2. Type 1 most commonly causes cold sores found on the mouth and is not usually sexually transmitted. Type 2 refers to the type that is sexually transmitted. HSV tends to start out as a single blister or multiple blisters that then come together. You may have no symptoms, or you may have burning and pain in the area, redness, or a vaginal discharge. It is important to see your doctor if you think you have an outbreak or an episode of herpes. There is currently no cure for HSV, but there are medications that are used to help shorten and decrease the outbreaks. If you are diagnosed with HSV, it is also recommended that you get screened for other sexually transmitted infections.

HUMAN IMMUNODEFICIENCY VIRUS (HIV)/ACQUIRED IMMUNODEFICIENCY SYNDROME AIDS

HIV is covered in this section, but I want to remind you that it is not just transmitted through sexual activity, it can also be transmitted via drug use and exposure to blood or blood products that were contaminated with HIV. Another way to contract it is from your mother in the womb. Some persons have HIV from birth and may not be aware that they have it. It is thought that one out seven new cases of HIV are in the adolescent group. This illness affects your body's ability to defend itself against other illnesses. HIV attacks and destroys the T helper cells (CD4) in the immune system, which can lead to AIDS. AIDS causes a group of illnesses to happen as a result of HIV's destruction of the immune system. When HIV is diagnosed, monitored, and treated early, it enables the person with the illness to have a better quality of life. It also enables them to educate others and take precautions or make decisions to help prevent others from becoming exposed, such as not having unprotected sex.

PELVIC INFLAMMATORY DISEASE (PID)

When an infection (such as gonorrhea or chlamydia) moves from the outside to the internal organs—the uterus, fallopian tubes, ovaries, or abdomen—this is referred to as inflammation of the pelvis. This infection can also go into the abdomen, causing one to become very sick.

PID is responsible for one to two out of every four sexually active adolescents with pelvic pain. This may be diagnosed if your pain is decreased with antibiotics. Sometimes your doctor may have to do surgery to see why you are having pain and to make sure you do not have inflammation in another part of your body, such as the appendix. During surgery, the doctor may see signs of infection in the pelvis and/ or signs of infection in the liver.

HUMAN PAPILLOMAVIRUS (HPV)

HPV is one of the most common STIs. There are many different types of HPV, which are currently divided into the high-risk types, (those known to cause cervical cancer) and low-risk types (those known to cause genital warts). Your body is often able to get rid of the HPV if you have a healthy immune system. The vaccine (see immunization section) also helps to protect you against HPV infections.

ZIKA

The Zika virus is transmitted mainly through bites from a mosquito (*Aedes aegypti*). However, the virus can also be transmitted through human to human contact, such as through sex or blood transfusions. When contracted during pregnancy, zika is linked to birth defects in the fetus's brain. Most people infected with Zika do not develop any symptoms, but about a quarter of those infected develop symptoms such as fever, redness, muscle aches, headache, other flu-like symptoms, conjunctivitis, ulceration of the mucous membranes, and digestive problems. If you have symptoms, they may last two to seven days.

HEPATITIS B AND HEPATITIS C

Hepatitis B and C are viruses that can affect the liver. They tend to be asymptomatic in adolescents. Sometimes the infections go away. If they become chronic they can cause liver damage. You can pass the virus to others through your bodily fluids and blood, so you should not share personal items with others. It you have a break in the skin, such as a cut, make sure it is covered.

PREVENTION OF SEXUALLY TRANSMITTED INFECTIONS

To prevent your exposure STIs, there are several options. The first is to avoid sexual activity. It's important to handle your body with care. The law prescribes the age you have to be to drink alcohol, drive, and to give permission to someone to have sex with you. Think about how important your body is and how much more sex could affect your body than alcohol or driving. Sexual activity comes with possible consequences and should be deferred until you understand these and are mature enough to deal with the results.

Another method of prevention is condoms. Condoms *help* to prevent STIs and unplanned pregnancies, but they do not remove the risk one hundred percent. They are much more affordable than a doctor's visit, antibiotics, surgery, or the pain of dealing with complications of uneducated or unwise choices.

1 Corinthians 7:1-2 (ESV)
Now concerning the matters about which you wrote: "It is good for a man not to have sexual relations with a woman." But because of the temptation to sexual immorality, each man should have his own wife and each woman her own husband.

Ephesians 5:3 (ESV)
But sexual immorality and all impurity or covetousness must not even be named among you, as is proper among saints.

1 Corinthians 6:18-20 (ESV)
Flee from sexual immorality. Every other sin a person commits is outside the body, but the sexually immoral person sins against his own body. Or do you not know that your body is a temple of the Holy Spirit within you,

whom you have from God? You are not your own, for you were bought with a price. So glorify God in your body.

SUMMARY POINTS

* Sex is an important topic to talk about with someone who is knowledgeable.
* Sexually transmitted infections are ones that can be transmitted sexually.
* If you are not sexually active, you are not at risk.
* If you are sexually active, it is important to be screened for sexually transmitted infections so that they can be found and treated.

CHAPTER 13

Contraception in Adolescence

❧

CONTRACEPTION (ALSO KNOWN AS FAMILY planning) should be considered during adolescence and young adulthood. Although you cannot predict the future, having knowledge about your options and the risks and benefits of each option will allow you to make wise decisions. For example, if you know you want to put off having children until your twenties or thirties or forties, you may choose to not become sexually active until this time, or you may take steps to avoid unintended pregnancy.

Contraception includes medication or devices that help prevent pregnancy. Contraception can also have other uses and benefits. We will review the risks and benefits of each one. You should get as much knowledge as you can so that you can figure out if you need contraception and, if you do, which method would be best for you.

Below is a table of the types of contraception and the risks and benefits of each method. Some of these methods are permanent, such as surgical sterilization. Some are long acting, such as the implant and the intrauterine device (IUD), and some serve for shorter periods of time, such as the oral contraceptive pills (OCPs), the hormonal ring, condoms, or the injection.

Table 7

Method of contraception	Protects against STIs (Yes or No)	Efficacy (%)	Advantages	Disadvantages
Abstinence	Yes	100	It is free. It protects you from STIs. There are no side effects.	None
Fertility awareness (Rhythm Method)	No	76	Free, no side effects.	You have to have regular cycles to be able to use this method.
Pull out/ withdrawal method (removal of penis before ejaculation)	No	72-96	It is free.	You have to rely on the male partner to participate. It is not as reliable, as sperm can be released before ejaculation.
Spermicide	No	72	It is affordable.	It has to be used correctly. Usage may be a challenge if you have a latex allergy.

Method of contraception	Protects against STIs (Yes or No)	Efficacy (%)	Advantages	Disadvantages
Condoms— Male condoms female condoms	Yes Yes	82 79	They are easily accessible, affordable, and easy to carry in a pocket or purse.	Have to be used correctly. Usage may be a challenge if you have a latex allergy. They may break if not used correctly. They do not help with menstrual cycle issues.
Injectables				
Depo-Provera	No	91	You do not have to remember to use it daily so you are less likely to miss an injection. It is reversible; its effects wear off once you stop using it. The effects begin with the first injection. One injection can prevent pregnancy. The side effects may decrease with time.	It may result in irregular bleeding, lack of menses, and weight gain. It may delay ovulation for up to a year after injection. Prolonged use may affect bone mineral density.

Method of contraception	Protects against STIs (Yes or No)	Efficacy (%)	Advantages	Disadvantages
Mesigyna®	No	94	You use if once a month. You still have a period. It is affordable.	Muscle injection that is given once a month.
Noristerat®	No	94	Once every 8 weeks. It is affordable.	Muscle injection. May cause bloating, headache, dizziness, nausea, reaction at the injection site, weight gain, irregular bleeding. Cannot be used if you have porphyria.

Method of contraception	Protects against STIs (Yes or No)	Efficacy (%)	Advantages	Disadvantages
Hormonal methods				
Oral contraceptive pill (OCP)	No	91–99	It is effective when used as directed. It may improve regularity of cycles. It may decrease pain associated with menses or endometriosis. You are in control and do not need you partner to take this. It decreases the risk of PID (Pelvic Inflammatory Disease). It decreases the risk of endometrial and ovarian cancer.	May cause nausea, vomiting, and breast tenderness first 2–3 cycles. Does not protect against STIs. Risk of clots in legs. Check with a physician to ensure that you are able to take them. Oral contraception is not recommended with certain medications or medical problems.

Method of contraception	Protects against STIs (Yes or No)	Efficacy (%)	Advantages	Disadvantages
Progesterone only pill	No	92-99	It may decrease bleeding during menses. It does not increase the risk of high blood pressure or heart disease. They can be taken while breastfeeding	You have to take it every day. You should take it around the same time each day. If you are more than 2–3 hours late, you have to use a backup method for the next 2 days. It may make changes to the menses such as irregular bleeding or spotting between cycles. It is not recommended if you have lupus. It may not work if you are taking HIV, seizure medication, narcolepsy, or tuberculosis medication.©

Method of contraception	Protects against STIs (Yes or No)	Efficacy (%)	Advantages	Disadvantages
				You may have short or heavy cycles, or no period at al.l Symptoms such as nausea, headache, and breast tenderness.
Patch	No	91	They have easy to follow instructions. They are small.	You must replace it weekly. It may cause skin reactions. It is visible.
Ring	No	91	They are easy to use. You do not need to think about contraception for a month.	Your body may expel it. You may have an increased risk of heart attack and stroke. It is a foreign body.
Emergency contraception (Morning after pill, Plan B, Ellaone)	No	91	It reduces the risk of pregnancy when started.	It may affect your cycle that month.

Method of contraception	Protects against STIs (Yes or No)	Efficacy (%)	Advantages	Disadvantages
Implants				
Implantable device (Jadelle®, Implanon®, Nexplanon®)	No	99	It is effective when used as directed. It may decrease frequency of periods. It may decrease pain with menses or endometriosis. It is effective for 3–5 years.	You may have breakthrough spotting. You may have pain with menses. An office procedure is required to place and remove it.
Nonhormonal Intrauterine Device (IUD)	No	99.2	It is effective for up to 7 years.	An office procedure is required to place and remove it. Discomfort may be experienced upon placement. It may increase bleeding with menses.

Method of contraception	Protects against STIs (Yes or No)	Efficacy (%)	Advantages	Disadvantages
Hormonal Intrauterine Device (IUD)	No	99 2	It is effective when used as directed, usually for 3-5 years. It may decrease heaviness and frequency of cycles. It may decrease pain associated with menses or endometriosis.	An office procedure is required to place and remove it. Discomfort may be experienced upon place-ment. It may decrease bleeding with menses. You may become amenorrheic

CONTRACEPTIVE METHODS

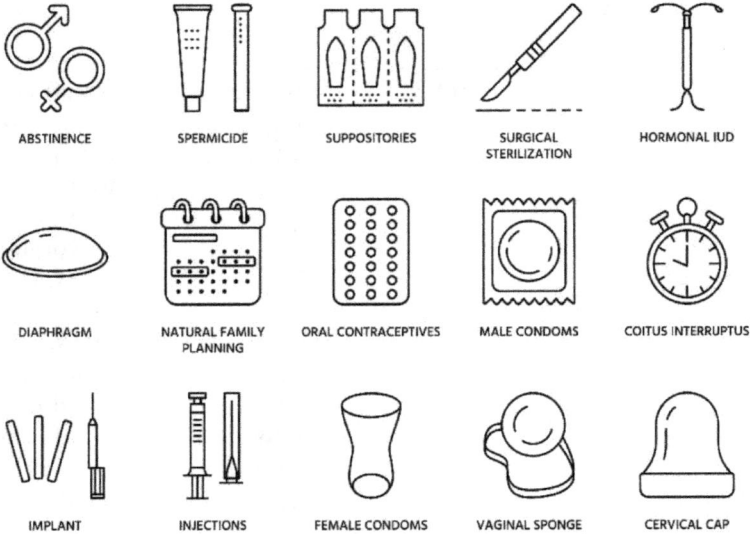

Figure 26. Contraceptive Methods

All the methods used for contraception are outlined above, but the most common methods used by adolescents include condoms and birth control pills (with the combined oral contraceptive being the most common type of birth control pill). Birth control pills have been around for more than fifty years. These are pills that you take every day or for twenty-one days in a month. They have hormones that prevent pregnancy. There are different types of birth control pills and your doctor can help you pick the one that would best suit you. Sometimes a lady has to try different types before finding the one that best suits her body.

If you have a history of clots in the legs or lungs, a disorder that increases your risk of clots (such as thrombophilia, factor V Leiden mutation, protein C or S deficiency, or antithrombin III), lupus, cyanotic heart disease, or pulmonary artery hypertension, you are not a candidate for the birth control pill. Just like any other medicine, the pill has risks and benefits.

Risks may include:

* Clots in legs and lungs (one in ten thousand ladies)
* Nausea
* Vomiting
* Headache
* Abdominal pain

Benefits may include:

* Decreased bleeding during periods
* Regulation of the period
* Decreased risk of cancers in endometrium
* Decreased risk of ovarian cancer

EMERGENCY CONTRACEPTION

This term refers to using contraception to prevent pregnancy within five days (one hundred and twenty hours) after unprotected sex. The two main ways to do this are by:

* Using pills designed for this purpose (the morning after pill)
* Inserting a copper intrauterine device (IUD)

Emergency contraception is not meant to be used as your only form of protection, nor should it be used regularly as it is not as effective as non-emergency (regular) contraceptive methods.

After taking emergency contraceptive pills, your period may come earlier or later. If you do not see a period within three weeks after using emergency contraception you should take a pregnancy test. If the test is negative, you can wait for your period. If it is positive, see your health-care provider.

SUMMARY POINTS

* As an adolescent or young adult, you have to take responsibility for your actions—especially decisions about when to have sex.
* Decide what your goals are for your sexual health.
* Let your behavior match. If you want to finish college or avoid pregnancy—do not engage in sexual activity—wait for marriage.
* If you are sexually active, take the time to review available contraceptive measures so that you can avoid STIs and unintended pregnancy.
* Your health-care provider will provide a safe, nonthreatening environment for you to discuss your concerns.
* Your health-care provider should listen to you and provide relevant information.
* Your health-care provider will discuss the advantages and disadvantages of your contraceptive options and recommend which one is best for you.

CHAPTER 14

Immunizations in Adolescence

❧

IMMUNIZATION IS THE PROCESS BY which a person is made resistant to an infectious disease. One way to have this happen is through vaccination. Vaccines are usually injections that encourage the body's own immune system to protect itself against subsequent disease. In other words, getting a vaccine for a certain disease will help prevent you from getting it..

The vaccines discussed below are given to adolescents and young adults. Your health-care provider may confirm that your immunizations are current (up-to-date). They may give advice about which ones are beneficial for you. Some important immunizations are:

- Tetanus-Diphtheria-Pertussis (Tdap) Booster
- Hepatitis A Vaccine
- Hepatitis B Vaccine
- Human Papillomavirus (HPV) Vaccine
- Influenza (Flu) Vaccine
- Meningococcal Vaccine

TETANUS-DIPHTHERIA-PERTUSSIS (TDAP) BOOSTER

This vaccine is given once every ten years. It is a combination vaccine that protects you against the bacterial illnesses: tetanus, diphtheria, and pertussis. They all can have serious effects on the body. Diphtheria can affect the heart, pertussis (whooping cough) can cause intense coughing, and tetanus can affect the brain and nervous system causing muscle spasms (e.g., lockjaw which prevents you from opening the mouth).

HEPATITIS A VACCINE

Hepatitis A is a foodborne or waterborne illness that causes inflammation of the liver and affects its ability to do its job. Symptoms include fever and jaundice (yellowing of the skin and/or eyes). The hepatitis A vaccine protects you from getting hepatitis A.

HEPATITIS B VACCINE

This vaccine is given to prevent the transmission of Hepatitis B. Hepatitis B is a viral infection of the liver. It may cause jaundice, fatigue, stomach trouble, or pain in the abdomen. It can be transmitted through sex, by being stuck with a contaminated needle, or an infected mother can pass it to her unborn child. The vaccine is given over two to three doses by way of an injection in the muscle.

HUMAN PAPILLOMAVIRUS (HPV) VACCINE

HPV is the virus that is responsible for genital warts and most cases of cervical cancer. Currently, there are two major brands of vaccine to protect against it—Cervarix and Gardasil. Depending on where you live, you may be familiar with one or the other. These vaccines reduce the chance of cervical cancer and genital warts by protecting you from some of the most common types of HPV. The vaccines are given at different times over a six-month period and involve two or three injections. Currently, the age that we start to give the vaccine is age 9.

Cervarix is designed to protect against HPV 16 and 18, which are responsible for most common causes of cervical cancer. Gardasil is now designed to protect against nine types of the HPV viruses,

(6,11,16,18,31,33,45,52, and 58). The most common side effects of the vaccine are dizziness, headache, fainting, fever, pain, muscle pain, redness at the injection site, and swelling. In rare cases, some ladies have an allergy to components of the vaccine.

INFLUENZA VACCINE

This vaccine is given once a year to protect you from the flu. The flu is a viral illness that spreads easily, especially in the first three to four days of becoming unwell. The flu virus also may change from year to year, so a new version of the vaccine is designed each year to protect against the most common versions of the virus for that year.

MEASLES, MUMPS, AND RUBELLA VACCINE

This vaccine protects you from measles, mumps, and rubella. These infections can all be harmful. Measles is a respiratory disease that is contagious and spreads through sneezing. Mumps can also cause serious complications and lives and reproduces in the respiratory tract. These infections can all cause fever, muscle aches, fatigue, headache, and swollen glands in the neck.

Although this vaccine is normally given in childhood, some teens and adolescents have not received it since some parents thought the vaccine was linked to autism. However, the latest research has shown that there is no link between autism and the MMR vaccine. If you were not vaccinated as a child, you can still be vaccinated as an adolescent, so speak to your health-care provider.

MENINGOCOCCAL VACCINE

This vaccine protects you from meningococcal disease, which is an illness caused by the bacteria *Neisseria meningitidis*. This infection affects the brain's lining and the spinal cord, causing fever, stiff neck, nausea, vomiting, sensitivity to light, confusion and/or headache. Since the symptoms can be similar to flu and other illnesses, it can be difficult to diagnose. Contracting the infection may have serious complications, including death. There are different types of meningococcal vaccine. Your health care provider can let you know which one would be right for you.

AFTER VACCINATION

The most common symptom that you may have after getting vaccinated is redness and soreness at the injection site. Some people may pass out (faint) when getting vaccinated, so you may be asked to lie down for a few minutes afterward. If you are concerned about a particular side effect, discuss it with your health-care provider. Many providers may also give you an information sheet on a particular vaccine, which will explain what side effects to watch for, if any.

SUMMARY POINTS

* Immunization is the process by which an injection is given to make a person resistant to contracting certain diseases.
* Immunizations are key to disease prevention.
* Your health-care provider will help you figure out which vaccines are recommended based on your age and activities.
* The most common side effect of a vaccine injection is redness and soreness at the injection site.
* Information sheets may be available about a vaccine, either before or after you receive it.

CHAPTER 15

Skin Problems in Adolescence

❦

Ezekiel 37:5–6 (NIV)
This is what the Sovereign Lord says to these bones: "I will make breath enter you, and you will come to life. I will attach tendons to you and make flesh come upon you and cover you with skin; I will put breath in you, and you will come to life. Then you will know that I am the Lord."

As a gynecologist, I do not manage skin problems, but patients often mention them during their visits with me. Adolescents are more likely than adults to have skin conditions, so we will review common skin concerns in your age group and some tips for caring for your skin.

You may find a pimple on your skin. This is one of the most common skin issues in your age group. Some of you may develop severe acne, which can leave scarring. This is called acne vulgaris. The main causes of acne are hormones and the genes that you have inherited from your parents. At puberty, the sebaceous (oil) glands around the hair follicles on your skin increase in size. Oil production increases and the ducts around the follicles get clogged. This is called acne. There are four common types of acne lesions. Knowing which type you have is the first step in figuring out what treatment is needed.

STAGES OF ACNE

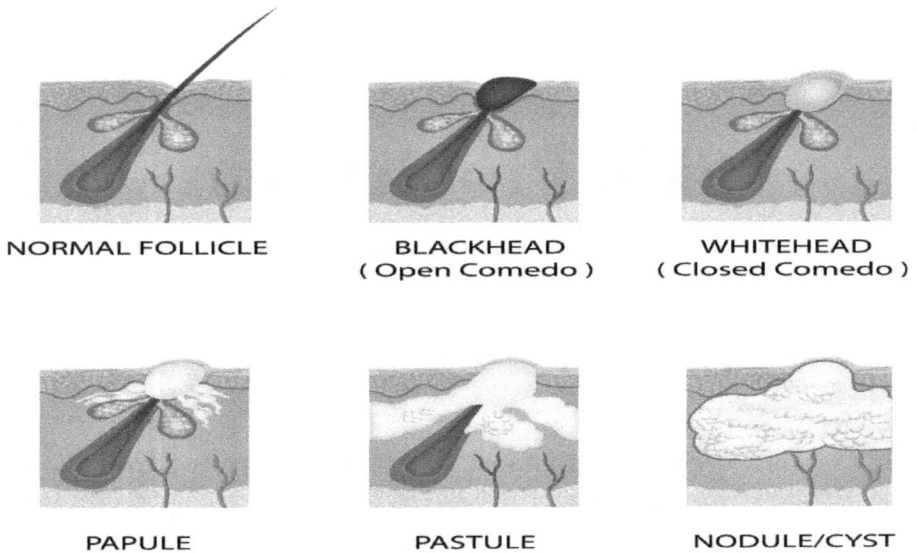

NORMAL FOLLICLE

BLACKHEAD
(Open Comedo)

WHITEHEAD
(Closed Comedo)

PAPULE

PASTULE

NODULE/CYST

Figure 27. Stages of acne

WHITEHEADS (CLOSED COMEDONES)

Closed Comedones appear as a small white bump or whitehead, which is the result of a plugged follicle underneath the skin. Whiteheads can sometimes be treated by an over-the-counter benzoyl peroxide cream or with prescription medications.

BLACKHEADS (OPEN COMEDONES)

Blackheads mostly show up on the face, nose, forehead, neck, chest, and back. These are caused by pores (tiny openings on the skin's surface) that are clogged by debris. They have a black center, which is the result of cells and oil in the follicle reacting with the air. To treat blackheads, gently clean your skin twice a day. If needed, you can sometimes open the clogged pores using products that contain benzoyl peroxide (a medication used to treat mild to moderate acne) four to seven times a week.

If you wear makeup, use non comedogenic face products, as they are less likely to cause blackheads to form.

PAPULES AND PUSTULES

Papules are small bumps on the skin that are inflamed. Pustules (pimples) are papules that are filled with pus. Topical medications (medications that are placed on the skin) such as those containing benzoyl peroxide or a retincid (which is usually prescribed) may help. If an oral antibiotic, oral contraceptive, or other prescription cream is needed, a skin doctor (dermatologist) or a gynecologist may prescribe them.

CYSTS OR NODULES

These are deeper, painful lesions that occur when there is an infection within the sebaceous gland. This infection causes the gland and the area around it to become abnormal as the infection spreads below the skin's surface. An oral antibiotic or other acne medication such as isotretinoin is often necessary to treat this problem and to help prevent scarring.

SKIN TREATMENT AND SKIN CARE

Most cases of pimples, blackheads, or whiteheads will clear up. But for some, acne can cause extremely painful, cyst-like lesions. Acne can continue for years, even into adulthood. But the good news is that most of the time, it will disappear when you reach your early twenties. Good skin starts from the inside and starts with good nutrition and adequate water intake.

Gently clean the skin at least twice daily. Do not irritate the skin with excessive scrubbing. Do not use products that include alcohol or other astringents or harsh detergents that can irritate the skin and constrict the pores, as these can make acne worse. Wear an oil-free or non-come-dogenic sunscreen when outdoors.

If you wear makeup, ensure it is non comedogenic and always remove it before going to bed using face wash or products that are designed to remove makeup.

Occasionally, nodules or deep bumps of acne persist. If this is the case, see a dermatologist. The dermatologist may prescribe topical antibiotics, oral antibiotics, or other acne medicines like isotretinoin. Your doctor will talk about the risks and benefits with you before you use them. For example, if you are sexually active, it is recommended to be on birth control with certain skin products, as they can be harmful if a lady gets pregnant while on the medication.

TIPS TO CARE FOR ACNE:

* Skin is affected by your diet, so make sure you are eating plenty of vegetables.
* Drink enough water and eat water-rich foods, as hydration is important.
* Keep all skin areas that are prone to acne very clean. Use soap and lots of water.
* Pat areas dry; do not rub the skin.
* Lukewarm water is best to avoid aggravating skin conditions. Water that is very hot or very cold is not recommended.
* See a dermatologist if you are concerned about your acne.

DERMATITIS/ECZEMA

This is also referred to as atopic dermatitis and is a common skin condition which may cause an itchy rash. This can be made worse by diet. Sometimes people with eczema may also have asthma. Avoiding the trigger or irritants can help those with dermatitis or eczema.

Pityriasis Versicolor (Shifting Clouds)

This is a common fungal infection that is caused by a type of yeast. The skin may appear scaly or pale and may become discolored with time. It is not harmful or contagious, but you can see your health-care provider, who may recommend some treatment.

Vitiligo

This is a disorder where patches of skin lose their pigment (color). Treatments are used to try to help the skin maintain its normal function, but many of them may not work.

Stretch Marks

These are common marks on the skin that can appear as you grow and put on weight. They can appear anywhere, but the most common areas are the breasts, stomach, thighs, arms, and backs of the legs. They are not harmful. They may be purple, pink, or silvery whitish in color and they tend to fade with time. There are creams and treatments to help them appear less noticeable, but they may not work. Laser treatments may help but may require multiple treatments and can be costly.

Summary Points

* You may notice skin issues during puberty and adolescences, such as blackheads and whiteheads.
* You may also have different skin conditions that are related to your immune system, such as eczema.
* You may need to see a dermatologist if the problems are not improving with routine skin care.

CHAPTER 16

Body Image and Eating Disorders

⤜⧉⤏

Song of Solomon 4:7 (NIV)
You are altogether beautiful, my darling; there is no flaw in you.

BODY IMAGE

Body image is how you feel about yourself when you look in the mirror. How you feel may be different from how you look. It is all about how you think you look. Your body image is a result of many influences, including your culture, your family, your emotions, your mood, and your hormones. Not feeling good about your body image puts you at risk for an eating disorder.

You can make a decision to have a positive body image and you can also encourage others to have a positive body image. Always love yourself and accept your body. Keep in mind the positive things about your body and pay attention to your own biases and beliefs about body size. Monitor your social media accounts and make sure that you expose yourself to all body types.

1 Corinthians 6:19-20 (ESV)
Or do you not know that your body is a temple of the Holy Spirit within you, whom you have from God? You are not your own, for you were bought with a price. So glorify God in your body.

Psalm 139:14 (ESV)
I praise you, for I am fearfully and wonderfully made. Wonderful are your works; my soul knows it very well.

EATING DISORDERS

An eating disorder affects all genders and ages, including adolescents. An eating disorder is a mental illness that results in an unhealthy relationship with food. In adolescence, you are constantly being bombarded with pressure about the way that you look by friends, family, and social media. These put you at risk for an eating disorder. You or someone you know may have an eating disorder, but there are many resources to help. The first step is recognizing there is an issue.

BULIMIA

Bulimia nervosa includes binge eating (filling up) and purging (cleaning out). Binge eating is when you eat more than the average person your age would eat. You may feel that you can't stop eating or that you can't control what or how much you eat. Then, to prevent weight gain, you may make yourself vomit, use laxatives, take water pills, or work out excessively. If you do this once a week for three months or more, then you may be diagnosed with bulimia. Self-evaluation is unduly influenced by body shape and weight. Sometimes, you may struggle with other mood disorders at the same time.

BINGE EATING DISORDER

This is an eating disorder that involves a loss of control of your eating. You may have a comorbid (another condition happening at the same time) mood disorder. This also puts you at risk for having issue with substances such as alcohol.

ANOREXIA

Anorexia nervosa is an eating disorder that involves weight loss (or lack of appropriate weight gain in your age group); problems maintaining an appropriate body weight for height, age, and stature; and, in many individuals, distorted body image. People with anorexia generally restrict the number of calories and the types of food they eat.

This disorder most frequently begins during adolescence. You cannot tell if a person is struggling with anorexia by looking at them. If you have anorexia nervosa, you would be cutting back on your food intake, which may cause low body weight for your age and gender. Even though you may already be underweight, you may be afraid of putting on weight or becoming fat.

AVOIDANT RESTRICTIVE FOOD INTAKE DISORDER

This disorder occurs when you are extremely picky, which may result in undernourishment as you limit the food types that you eat.

GET HELP

Once you recognize a problem, get help. Many online resources are available. Use a search engine to look for the following organizations.

* Academy of Eating Disorders
* National Eating Disorder Association
* Association of Anorexia Nervosa and Related Disorders
* Binge Eating Disorder Association

There are also books that may be helpful, such as "It's Not About Food: End Your Obsession with Food and Weight" by Carol Emery Normandi and "Not All Black Girls Know How to Eat: A Story of Bulimia" by Stephanie Covington Armstrong.

SUMMARY POINTS

- Eating disorders are serious health issues that can result in death.
- We all come in different shapes and sizes. You are beautiful. Embrace who you are.
- You should aim to eat healthy and be healthy.
- If you are struggling in this area, get professional help.

SCRIPTURES

1 Corinthians 10:31 (ESV)
So, whether you eat or drink, or whatever you do, do all to the glory of God.

2 Timothy 1:7 (ESV)
For God gave us a spirit not of fear but of power and love and self-control.

Proverbs 25:16 (ESV)
If you have found honey, eat only enough for you, lest you have your fill of it and vomit it.

Proverbs 23:19-21(ESV)
Hear, my son, and be wise, and direct your heart in the way. Be not among drunkards or among gluttonous eaters of meat, for the drunkard and the glutton will come to poverty, and slumber will clothe them with rags.

Proverbs 11:14(ESV)
Where there is no guidance, a people falls, but in an abundance of counselors there is safety.

CHAPTER 17

Obesity in Adolescence

❧

3 John 1:2 (ESV)
Beloved, I pray that all may go well with you and that you may be in good health, as it goes well with your soul.

Obesity is defined as being overweight. This is an issue that affects many young people and can impact their lives now and in the future. Obesity increases your chance of getting diabetes, heart disease, and cancer. You can use the body mass index (BMI) to figure out if your weight is healthy for your height. To do this, you divide your weight by your height. Once your BMI has been calculated, you can determine which group you fall into. For example, if your BMI is 18.5-

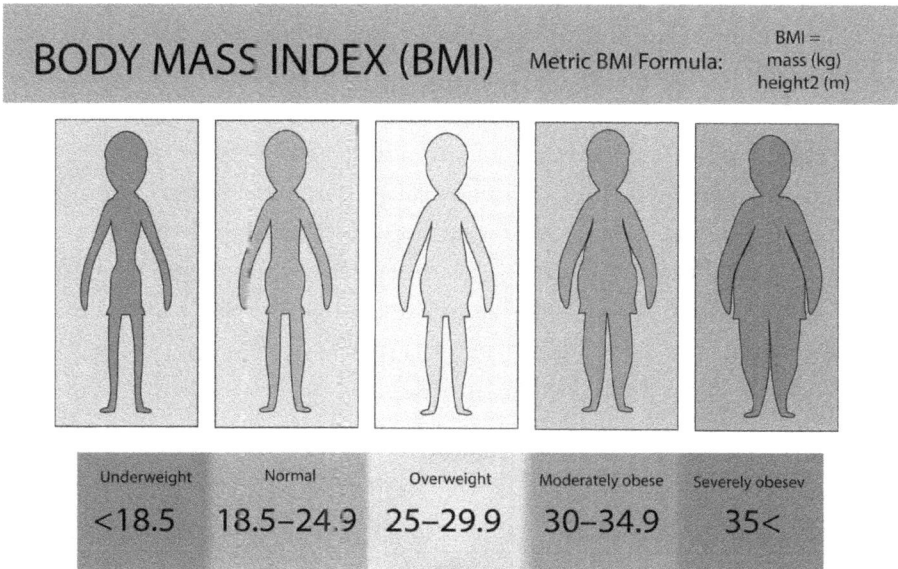

Figure 28. Obesity mass index

The best way to maintain a healthy weight is to have a balanced diet of vitamins, protein, fruits, vegetables, and grains. You do not have to give up all the things that you love. However, it is good to eat things in moderation. Look for a healthy alternative to unhealthy snacks. For example, nuts or fresh fruit instead of doughnuts.

Eat what you need. Do not overeat. Instead of eating what you can tolerate, eat until you are close to full. Consider only eating when you are hungry, rather than eating because it is time to eat. Eating high-fiber foods such as oatmeal and vegetables (like broccoli and cauliflower) can help you feel full longer. Monitor the amount of carbohydrates that you take in from foods like bread and potatoes. Monitor the amount of juice that you drink as it contains high amounts of sugar.

Water is important for the body. In fact, the body is made up mostly of water. Water can help flush out toxins (harmful substances) from the body.

Exercise is important in adolescence. Teenagers need at least 30-60 minutes of moderate to vigorous physical activity each day to maintain good health and fitness while you are growing. Exercise may be aerobic, muscle strengthening, and/or bone strengthening. Exercise has benefits that you see immediately (short term) and some that you will see in the future (long term). Short term it can make you feel happier, increase your energy, and help you sleep better. Long term benefits include that it decreases your risk of chronic diseases such as type II diabetes, high cholesterol, and cancer, and that it can increase your life span. Exercise is thought to help both the physical body the brain. For example, it helps you have better memory, reduces your risk of depression, and may help you do better in your academic studies.

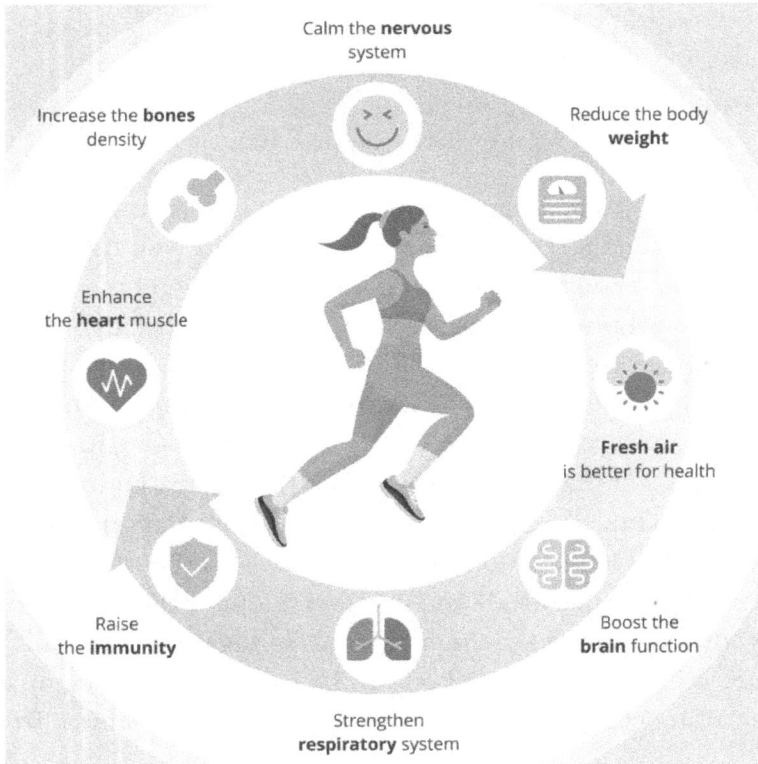

Figure 29. Benefits of exercise

Summary Points

* Make healthy eating choices as much as possible, such as fruits, vegetables, and high-protein foods.
* Eat until you are close to full.
* Eat only when you are hungry.
* Drink plenty of water and avoid sugary drinks and alcohol.
* Exercise.

Proverbs 25:16 (NIV)
If you find honey, eat just enough—too much of it, and you will vomit.

Philippians 3:19 (NIV)
Their destiny is destruction their god is their stomach, and their glory is in their shame. Their mind is set on earthly things.

Proverbs 25:28 (ESV)
A man without self-control is like a city broken into and left without walls.

CHAPTER 18

Cancer in Adolescence

❦

Proverbs 17:22 (NIV)
A cheerful heart is good medicine, but a crushed spirit dries up the bones.

Unfortunately, cancer can happen in young people too. Cancer is the most common cause of disease-related death in adolescents and young adults in high-income countries. Cancer happens when cells that make up the body do not stop growing when they are supposed to. This creates a problem as they take over an area and then move to other parts of the body (metastasis). Sometimes this can be brought under control or prevented with effective treatment.

If you are not feeling well, it's important to bring that to the attention of the person taking care of you. You are the best person to stand up for yourself. You may recognize that something is not normal before anyone else does. *If* you are given a diagnosis of malignancy (cancer), educate yourself and your family about the disease and treatment options. Ask questions about the risks, benefits, and success rate of each treatment offered. Ask about other things that you can do to improve outcomes too, such as diet changes.

LYMPHOMA

This is a cancer of the blood that affects the white cells called lymphocytes. This is one of the most common types of cancer in adolescents and young adults. There are two types of lymphoma: Hodgkin's or Non-Hodgkin's. The treatment and treatment outcomes are influenced by the person's overall health and stage of illness. If you were diagnosed with this, your health-care provider would refer you to a specialist with expertise in this area.

LEUKEMIA

This is a cancer that affects the white cells that are responsible for fighting infection in the body. When a person has leukemia, their body produces white cells that are abnormal and cannot carry out their normal function of fighting infection. As a result of this illness, the chance of infection is increased. Anything that may affect your immune system, such as radiation, chemotherapy, or a family history of this illness or other inherited disorders can increase your chances of getting leukemia. There are different types of leukemia. Many teens and young adults are successfully treated for this.

PHYLLODES TUMOR

This can be noncancerous or cancerous and comes from the lobular connective tissue in the breast. This is the most common form of breast cancer in adolescents. It is more common in some populations than others. If you have a lump in your breast that is growing quickly, please see your health-care provider right away.

TUMORS OF THE OVARY

Patients with an ovarian tumor may have no symptoms or they may have pain, nausea, vomiting, an increase in the size of the abdomen, or changes to their period. These tumors are divided into different groups depending on the tissue that they started from and what they are made of. Some of the more common categories in adolescents are as follows:

* Malignant germ cell tumors:
  o Immature teratoma
  o Endodermal sinus tumors

* Non-germ cell tumors:
  o Sex cord-stromal tumors
  o Granulosa cell tumor

Ultrasound is used to help make the diagnosis prior to removal of the tumor. Blood work, including tumor markers (blood tests that may be elevated), are also measured. Your procedure may be done by a gynecologic oncologist (a gynecologist that specializes in the management of cancer in females). They will also advise you if additional treatment is needed post procedure and tell you the risk of the tumor coming back.

METASTATIC CANCER IN THE OVARY

Cancers from other parts of the body such as gastric cancer or lymphomas can move to the ovaries.

BREAST CANCER

Breast cancer is unlikely in your age group. However, secretory carcinoma is the most common type of breast cancer found in adolescents, and it tends to have an excellent outcome once it's found and treated. Other cancers, such as malignant cystosarcoma phyllodes, lymphoma, neuroblastomas, sarcoma, rhabdomyosarcoma, and acute leukemia may also cause lumps in the breast.

METASTATIC CANCER IN THE BREAST

You may have a blood cancer or muscle cancer that can move to the breast. If the cancer starts from another location and then moves to the breast, it is called metastatic.

FERTILITY POST TREATMENT

If you have cancer and you have to have treatment, it may affect your ability to have children in the future. Ask your cancer doctor about this issue. There is probably a good chance that they have a solution in mind and can put you in touch with a physician who can carry out that solution. Some solutions that may be considered include:

* Ovarian tissue preservation
* Oocytes preservation
* Uterus transplantation

SUMMARY POINTS

* Cancers are not common in adolescents, but they do happen.
* There are fertility options for the future; make sure to discuss these with your health-care provider.
* Continue to maintain a positive attitude as you work through this.
* Meditate on the scriptures provided below.

SCRIPTURES

Isaiah 38:16 (NIV))
Lord, by such things people live; and my spirit finds life in them too. You restored me to health and let me live.

Isaiah 41:10 (NIV)

So do not fear, for I am with you; do not be dismayed, for I am your God. I will strengthen you and help you. I will uphold you with my righteous right hand.

Philippians 4:6 (NIV)

Do not be anxious about anything, but in every situation, by prayer and petition, with thanksgiving, present your requests to God.

CHAPTER 19

Other Issues in Adolescence

❦

PLASTIC SURGERY

Plastic surgery is used to modify an area of the body that may not be normal or may be normal, but that the person is unsatisfied with. It is not recommended that adolescents have cosmetic surgery, as the body changes throughout this period.

URINARY TRACT INFECTION/BLADDER INFECTION

The bladder is responsible for holding your urine (pee). If bacteria get in the urine, depending on how far up the urinary tract it goes, determines the name and severity of the infection. If it is in the area of the tube that leads to the outside (urethra) then you have a urethritis. If the infection travels up to the bladder, you will have an infection called cystitis. If you have a urinary tract infection, you may have to urinate more frequently and have pain when you pee. You also may feel like you can't empty your bladder all the way or have blood in your urine. You may have back pain and low-grade fever. Your symptoms can be mild or severe.

Pyelonephritis (Kidney Infection)

If the bladder infection moves to your kidney, this may cause flank pain, chills, vomiting, and muscle aches. You may have to be admitted to the hospital.

Prolapsed Urethra/Urethrocele

Prolapsed urethra is a condition where the inner lining of the end of the tube that you urinate from protrudes a bit. This area can sometimes be painful and may bleed a little or swell.

Urethral Diverticulum

This is when a sac forms under the urethra. This may at times fill with urine or become infected (filled with pus). This may cause pain or there may be dribbling when you urinate.

Kidney Stones

These are not common in adolescents and young adults. A stone is hard material formed in the kidneys or urinary tract that can cause pain in the groin or back and comes and goes (colicky pain). Kidney stones can also cause blood in the urine.

Accidental Genital Trauma

Accidental injury to the genital region can happen if you fall across a blunt or sharp object such as a bicycle bar or the edge of the tub or are in a car accident. These accidents may result in bruising or a cut in the genital areas or bleeding. You may have swelling and pain that could stop you from being able to pee. If this happens, you should be evaluated by a health-care provider to ensure that no long-term damage has been done to the area. Sometimes the area has to be examined in theater (a place where surgery is done) with anesthesia so that the area may be completely evaluated and any injury that requires repair can be fixed.

SUMMARY POINTS

* Leave elective plastic surgery procedures until you have completed your growth and development.
* Problems with the bladder or kidney may cause pain, so seek help.
* If you have an infection, follow the instructions given by your health-care provider so that the infection does not worsen.
* If you have an accident that affects the genitals, do not be embarrassed. Let your health-care provider know so they can make sure that everything is okay.

CHAPTER 20

Mental Health in Adolescence

~~~

Proverbs 12:25 (NIV)
Anxiety weighs down the heart, but a kind word cheers it up.

Mental health is so important. Your mind enables you to function. Just as you can have changes in other parts of the body, you can have some changes in the mind as well. If you feel that something is not right with your thoughts, do not try to handle it by yourself. It is a challenging position to be in. There is usually at least one person in your life you can confide in and who may be able to give you guidance. If not, do not hesitate to discuss it with your health-care provider.

MOOD SWINGS

Mood swings occur in adolescence, as many hormonal changes and psychosocial changes occur during this time. It may be difficult to differentiate between what is thought to be a normal change compared to an abnormal change. It is a good idea to discuss this with a health-care provider. They can say whether what you are experiencing is normal or not.

Premenstrual Syndrome (PMS)

This a condition where you have behavioral, emotional, and psychological symptoms that are linked to the luteal phase of your cycle. Young ladies may have symptoms about a week or two before their period. These symptoms may include:

* A low mood
* Irritability
* Hunger
* Joint pain,
* Headache
* Constipation
* Breast tenderness
* Acne

These symptoms can be mild or intense. Symptoms usually improve after the period and before ovulation. It is recommended that you keep track of the symptoms for two months and look at the timing of them and compare them to where you are in your menstrual cycle (see chapter on phases of menstrual cycle).

Please record any symptoms that you have. Experiencing one or more of the symptoms for three consecutive cycles would mean that you may have PMS, so your record of them may be important and can help you and your provider make a diagnosis.

If you have these symptoms, please discuss them with your health-care provider. Sometimes your health-care provider may recommend review by a mental health specialist, supplements such as calcium, or oral contraceptive to assist with the symptoms.

PREMENSTRUAL DYSPHORIC DISORDER (PMDD)

We do not understand the exact cause of premenstrual dysphoric disorder (PMDD), but it may be due to a decrease in a hormone called serotonin, which plays a part in mood. If a young lady has severe symptoms five to eleven days before her period, it is of concern.

DYSTHYMIA (PERSISTENT DEPRESSIVE DISORDER)

If you have dysthymia, you may have one or more of the following:

* Depressed or irritable mood for most of the day for more than a year.
* Never without the symptoms below for more than two months.
* Two or more of the symptoms of major depression, such as:
* Persistent feelings of sadness, hopelessness or helplessness
* Having low self-esteem/feeling inadequate
* Poor appetite or overeating
* Feelings of wanting to die/suicidal thoughts or attempts
* Difficulty with relationships
* Sleep disturbances (sleeping too much or not sleeping enough)
* Changes in appetite or weight
* Decreased energy
* Difficulty concentrating or making decisions
* Irritability, hostility, or aggression
* Frequent physical complaints (for example, headache, stomachache, or fatigue)
* Running away or threatening to run away from home
* Loss of interest in usual activities or activities once enjoyed
* Hypersensitivity to failure or rejection

DEPRESSION

Depression is when you have sadness and loss of interest or pleasure that is not linked to any medical reason. This may have physical and emotional symptoms that last for more than two weeks. Although the table below is intended to help share some of the symptoms that may be associated with depression, it is important that if you think you have this condition, you seek professional help. Talk about it with your guardian and your health-care provider.

Some risk factors (things that increase your chance of having it) are

* A family history of depression
* Being female
* Obesity
* Puberty
* Other psychological disorders such as anxiety and learning disorders
* Sleep disturbances

If you are depressed, you will have five or more of the following symptoms:

Table 8

Symptoms of Depression	
Physical Symptoms	*Emotional Symptoms*
Weight loss or Weight gain	Sad or anxious mood
Increase or Decrease in Appetite	Restlessness, irritability
Fatigue	Increased tearfulness
Back pain	Lack of self-worth or guilt
Headaches	Loss of interest in activities that
Oversleeping or not sleeping	you usually enjoy

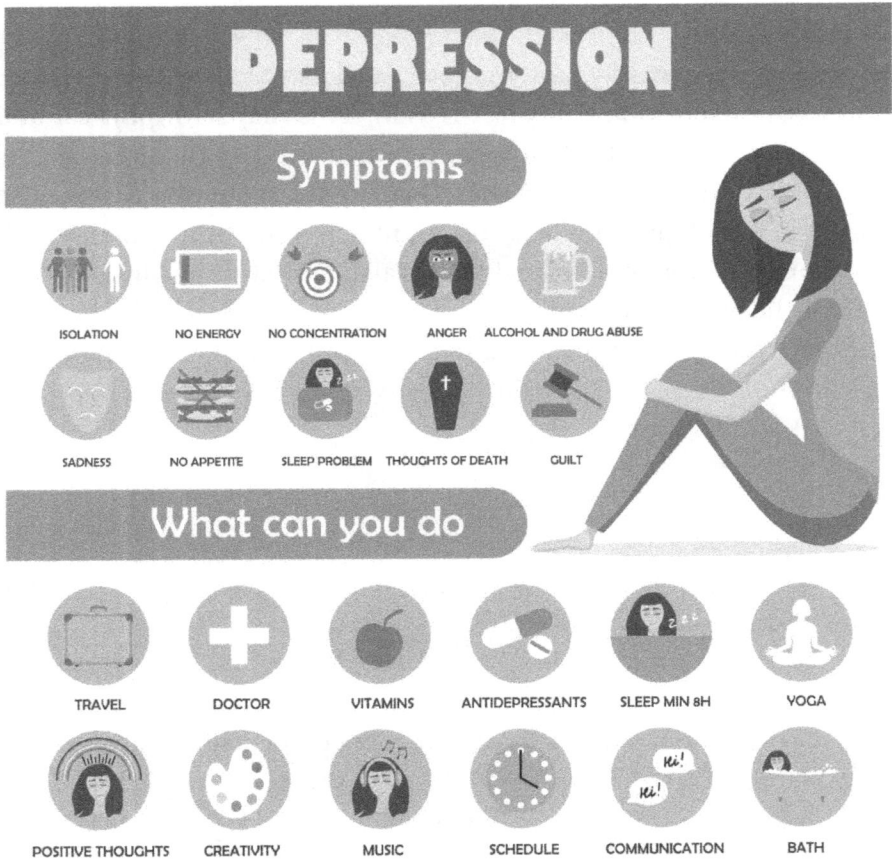

Figure 30. Depression

SUICIDE

Suicide is when you intentionally take your own life. Suicide is one of the top causes of death for adolescents. Suicide can be prevented in many cases. You can help to prevent it too. If you or a friend has thought of hurting yourself or themselves, address is right away. Let someone know so they can help you locate the correct resources to help. DO NOT try to deal with it by yourself. Sometimes you may have medical problems or mental health issues that can increase your risk of thinking about suicide. If you have a family history of suicide or have attempted suicide in the past, this also increases your risk. But, an increased risk does not mean you have to fall victim to suicide. It means that you have to pay attention to any changes in your emotions and avoid situations that make you feel life is not worth living.

Summary Points

* Having a mind that is healthy is as important as having a healthy body.
* There are normal emotional changes that occur with puberty and young adulthood which may result in mood swings.
* There are mental illnesses such as premenstrual dysmorphic disorder and depression that require additional help.
* It is important to establish a relationship with a good support person.
* If you have suicidal thoughts, please let an adult know.

Scriptures for Encouragement During Tough Times

Psalm 30:11 (ESV)
You have turned for me my mourning into dancing; you have loosed my sackcloth and clothed me with gladness.

Isaiah 41:10 (ESV)
Fear not, for I am with you; be not dismayed, for I am your God; I will strengthen you, I will help you, I will uphold you with my righteous right hand.

Matthew 11:28 (ESV)
Come to me, all who labor and are heavy laden, and I will give you rest.

Proverbs 3:5–6 (ESV)
Trust in the Lord with all your heart, and do not lean on your own understanding. In all your ways acknowledge him, and he will make straight your paths.

Psalm 143:7–8 (ESV)
Answer me quickly, O Lord! My spirit fails! Hide not your face from me, lest I be like those who go down to the pit. Let me hear in the morning of your steadfast love, for in you I trust. Make me know the way I should go, for to you I lift up my soul.

1 Peter 5:7 (ESV)
Cast all your anxieties on him, because he cares for you.

Philippians 4:6–7 (ESV)
Do not be anxious about anything, but in everything by prayer and supplication with thanksgiving let your requests be made known to God. And the peace of God, which surpasses all understanding, will guard your hearts and your minds in Christ Jesus.

Psalm 23:4 (ESV)
Even though I walk through the valley of the shadow of death, I will fear no evil, for you are with me; your rod and your staff, they comfort me.

Romans 8:28 (ESV)
And we know that for those who love God all things work together for good, for those who are called according to his purpose.

Psalm 9:9 (ESV)
The Lord is a stronghold for the oppressed, a stronghold in times of trouble.

QUESTIONS THAT YOU MAY HAVE

What age do I need to see a gynecologist?
Your first visit with a gynecologist (a doctor who specializes in female health) should be between the ages of twelve and fifteen. This gives you a chance to talk about the changes that are happening in your body. It also gives the doctor an opportunity to check that you are developing normally.

My breasts are uneven—is this normal?
In some ladies the breasts may be different in size or shape. Some of these differences may be slight, but some may be due to abnormal causes. So, if you feel that your breasts are uneven, please review this with your health-care provider.

What can I use for period pain?
What you use for pain depends on how bad the pain is and what works for you. Some ladies use heating pads and rest. Other ladies require over-the-counter medications such as Motrin or acetaminophen. Occasionally medication prescribed by a physician is required.

My friend said she had to go on birth control to help with her period pain; do I need to do that too?
If you have primary dysmenorrhea, birth control may help. Your health-care provider and guardians may opt to try you on medication that decreases pain before or along with birth control.

Can birth control help with acne?
In some ladies, the hormones in birth control may help with the acne.

What are menstrual cups made of?
A menstrual cup is placed in the vagina during your period and is made of medical grade silicone (tested for use in the body).

What does MHM stand for?
MHM stands for menstrual hygiene management. This covers how you will handle your period. There is a day, May 28, dedicated to this topic. In some countries, there are things that a young lady may be stopped from doing during her period. This may make it difficult for her to manage her period safely, which includes having material to absorb or collect the blood, having soap and water to wash, and being able to get rid of materials used during menstruation.

You may consider having a little cosmetic bag or pouch that you put your products in. You may also want to keep a change of underwear on hand in there, in case you soil your clothes while at school or work (an accident). If your periods are heavy, consider putting a dark colored sheet over your bed. That way if you have spillage you do not have to make up the whole bed.

How do I avoid body odor?
Tips to help prevent body odor include taking regular showers or bathing. Make sure to wash areas like under the arms, between your legs, the belly button, behind the ears, and your feet. Be sure to brush your teeth, tongue, and gums. Watch your diet and eat healthy foods as this can affect how you smell. Doing your laundry so that your clothes are clean, wearing breathable fabrics, and using hypoallergenic antiperspirants, deodorants, or natural methods will help to decrease or stop body odor.

How often should menstrual pads be changed?
Pads should be changed at least three times a day, if not more.

How often should tampons be changed?
A tampon should be changed every four to six hours. Make sure you use the tampon that is appropriate for your flow. For example, use a super tampon on heavy flow days and a light or regular tampon for regular flow days.

Should I pick a plastic or cardboard applicator for my tampon?
It is your choice. The cardboard applicator is more environmentally friendly, but the plastic applicator may be easier to use. There are also applicators that you can purchase that are reusable.

I am a virgin. Can I use a tampon?
You can use a tampon depending on the type of hymen you have. Discuss this with your health-care provider.

How do I know when to change a tampon?
You can change it on a schedule, or if you tug lightly on the string and the tampon slides out easily, then it is most likely soaked and time to change it.

Why do I still leak with my tampon or pad?
If you are leaking around your tampon, check that it is one that fits your body. You may also want to change it more frequently. Sometimes you can use both a tampon and a pad if necessary.

Where can you safely and hygienically dispose of pads?
Pads should be thrown away in disposal bins, pit latrines, or should be burned. Do not throw pads into toilets as this may cause problems with the plumbing system.

What do I do if I have a lost tampon?
If you cannot find the strings, you may have to see a health-care provider who can help you remove it. The tampon can only go in so far and can be retrieved by a health-care provider with the correct knowledge and instruments.

Is it okay to sleep with a tampon in?
It is thought to be safe as long as you are sleeping less than eight hours. I, as a gynecologist, avoid recommending it to adolescents as sometimes you sleep more hours than usual and may be reluctant to get up to change it.

My period started last year. Is it normal that I am not seeing my period every month?
Yes, in the first few years when the period starts, it may not come every month. However, if you are sexually active and you miss your period you should take a pregnancy test.

When will my period stop?
The average age that a period stops forever is fifty-one. This is called menopause. In rare cases, adolescents may have their period stop because they have ovarian insufficiency. If your health-care provider is concerned about this, they may order some testing to check for genetic, autoimmune, metabolic, or infectious processes.

What if I miss a birth control pill?
You should consult your health-care provider. Many of the packages have instructions on what to do depending on where you are in the pill pack and the number of pills that you have missed. For example, if you miss two pills at the beginning of the pack, you may be advised to take the two pills as soon as you realize that you have missed a day.

I have not had penetrative sex, but I have had oral sex. Can I get pregnant or get sexually transmitted infections?
No, you cannot get pregnant from oral sex. But you can pick up sexually transmitted infections.

I have not had sex, but we are rubbing our private parts on each other (male and female). Can I get pregnant?

Yes, you can get pregnant. Any action that possibly puts semen close the vagina, including dry rubbing, vaginal, or anal sex can result in a pregnancy.

I am having a vaginal discharge—is this normal?

If you have a discharge from the vagina, pay attention to the color, the smell, and any other symptoms such as fever, pain, burning, or itching and any soaps or detergents you've used. Sometimes a vaginal discharge is a normal part of the menstrual cycle. Sometimes the discharge is the result of a noninfectious cause, such as yeast or bacterial vaginosis. However, you should not try to self-diagnose (identify a medical condition yourself). You should seek professional help. If you are sexually active, the cause may be an infection such as gonorrhea, chlamydia, or trichomoniasis.

I have missed a period. Does that mean I am pregnant?

No, it does not mean that you are pregnant if you are not sexually active. If you are sexually active, then, yes, you may be pregnant. If you've been sexually active and missed a period, see your health-care provider and take a pregnancy test.

Can using a powder cause cancer?

Yes, we are concerned that powder use may be linked to ovarian cancer, so we do not recommend usage in the genital area.

Should I douche?

Douching is not recommended. The vagina has different types of bacteria that keep it healthy and douching may change that balance.

Can I use douching to avoid getting pregnant?
No. Douching is not an effective form of contraception. There are many more reliable methods. If you have had unprotected sex, you can take emergency contraception within seventy-two hours. This would be more effective than douching.

I have not seen my period yet—does that mean I cannot get pregnant?
No, it does not. You can still get pregnant, even if you are not seeing a period or do not have regular periods, if you are sexually active. The best way to prevent pregnancy is abstinence.

I am having pain in the stomach—should I be worried?
If you are having pain, you should let a parent or guardian know. There are many things that can cause pain; some of them are not serious and some are. If you have pain and, especially, if it is not getting better, talk about it with your health-care provider.

Adolescence is a tough time, but it can also be a rewarding time. It can include some of the best memories and experiences of your life. I, as an adult, reflect and tell stories from my adolescence and my young adult years. When you think back on times and moments that you can remember, you should be able to laugh or smile.

I get it. I understand. You may feel overwhelmed and unprepared at times. But information and education can help to ease the way forward. Take time to learn about yourself. Take time to build relationships— your relationship with God, your relationship with yourself, your relationship with your parents, your relationships with your peers.

Make wise choices. If you are not sure about something, get the appropriate advice and information from a reliable source. There is only one you! We all have gifts that have been given to us by God. You have so many gifts and talents to share. Take time to find out what your gift is. Take time to dream! Anyone who knows you has been given a privilege and honor. So take the time to get to know who you are. Be you! Understand your purpose! Live your life to the fullest! Progress through your adolescence into young adulthood with confidence.

3 John 2 (KJV)
Beloved, I wish above all things that thou mayest prosper and be in health, even as thy soul prospereth.

Pages for Your Thoughts or Questions

INDEX

Note: Page numbers followed by *t* indicate tables and *f* indicate figures.

A

Abscess: Bartholin's glands, 62; breast, 25–26

Abstinence. *See* Sexual abstinence

Abuse: physical, 74, 74*f*; screening, 73–74; sexual, 62, 74

Academy of Eating Disorders, 110

Accessory breast tissue, 22–23

Accidental genital trauma, 122–123

Acetaminophen, 131

Acne, 103, 131; blackheads, 104–105; care, tips, 106; papules and pustules, 105; skin treatment and skin care, 105–106; stages of, 104*f*; whiteheads, 104

Acne vulgaris, 103

Acquired immune deficiency syndrome (AIDS), 83

Adolescence, 3

Adolescent growth spurt, 35–36

Adrenarche, 28

Adrenocorticotropic hormone (ACTH), 15

Alcohol, 76; and bone health, 37

Allergic contact dermatitis, and vulvovaginitis, 61

Alopecia, 34

Amenorrhea, 49; chronic illnesses, eating disorders, and obesity, 52; constitutional delay of puberty, 49; genetic causes of, 50; and hormonal issues, 51; and pituitary mass, 52; and pregnancy, 50; and primary ovarian insufficiency, 51–52; secondary, 52; structural issues with female reproductive system, 50–51

Androgen insensitivity syndrome, 50

Anorexia nervosa, 110

Anterior (front) lobe, 15–16

Anus, 12

Association of Anorexia Nervosa and Related Disorders, 110

Atopic dermatitis, 106

Avoidant restrictive food intake disorder, 110

B

Bacterial infections: sexually transmitted infections, 81–82, 83–84; vaccines, 99–100, 101–102; and vulvar ulcers, 64; and vulvovaginitis, 60

Bartholin's glands, 12; cysts/abscess, 62

Benzoyl peroxide, 104, 105

Biannual exam, 8

Binge eating disorder, 109

Phyllodes tumor, 26, 117

Physical abuse, 74, 74*f*

Physical changes, and puberty, 2

Pimples, 103, 105

Pituitary gland, 15; hormones, 15–16, 16*f*; mass in, 52

Pityriasis versicolor, 107

Plan B pill, 93*t*

Plastic applicators, tampon, 133

Plastic surgery, 121

Polycystic ovary syndrome (PCOS), 51, 67–70, 68*f*; effects of, 69*t*; symptoms, 69*f*

Pornography, 77

Powder, and ovarian cancer, 135

Pregnancy, 80; and amenorrhea, 50; contraception (*see* Contraception); and irregular periods, 135; and missed periods, 135; and non-penetrative sex, 135; and oral sex, 134

Premenstrual dysphoric disorder (PMDD), 52–53, 126

Premenstrual syndrome (PMS), 52–53, 125

Primary dysmenorrhea, 54, 70, 131

Primary ovarian insufficiency, 51–52

Progesterone, 19

Progesterone only pills, 92–93*t*

Prolactin, 16

Prolapsed urethra. *See* Urethral prolapse

Prolonged menses, 58

Prostaglandins, 43

Pubarche, 28

Puberty, 1, 2–3; constitutional delay of, 49; and emotions, 2, 5; and hair, 29; hypothalamic-pituitary axis, 44; physiology of, 44–45

Pubic hair, staging, 29*t*

Pull out/withdrawal method, 88*t*

Purulent nipple discharge, 25

Pustules, 105

Pyelonephritis, 122

R

Reproductive endocrinologist, 50

Reproductive system: external organs, 10*f*, 11–12; internal organs, 12, 13–14, 13*f*; reproductive cycle, 44*f*; structural issues with, 50–51

Ring, contraceptive, 93*t*

S

Scabies, vulva, 63

Scoliosis, 39, 39*f*

Screening, 7, 73; abuse, 73–74, 74*f*; alcohol, 76; bone health, 38–39; bullying, 75–76; drugs, 77; pap test, 73; pornography, 77; sexual harassment, 76; smoking, 76–77

Secondary amenorrhea, 52

Secondary dysmenorrhea, 54, 55, 70

Self-identity, and puberty, 2

Serotonin, 126

Sex, 79–80; definition of, 80; oral, 134; types of, 80

Sex hormones, 44

Sexual abstinence, 80, 85, 88*t*, 136

Sexual abuse: screening, 74; and vulvovaginitis, 62

Sexual harassment, 76

Sexually transmitted diseases (STDs). *See* Sexually transmitted infections (STIs)

Sexually transmitted infections (STIs), 80, 81, 82–83; chlamydia, 82; gonorrhea, 81–82; hepatitis B and hepatitis C, 84–85; herpes simplex virus, 82–83; HIV/AIDS, 83; human papillomavirus, 84; and oral sex, 134; pelvic inflammatory disease, 83–84; prevention of, 85; syphilis, 82; trichomoniasis, 82; Zika virus, 84

Shaving, 29*t*, 32

Sitz baths, 61

Skene's gland, 12

Skin problems, 103; acne, 103–106, 104*f*; dermatitis/eczema, 106; pityriasis versicolor, 107; stretch marks, 107; vitiligo, 107

Smoking, 75–77; and bone health, 37

Speculum exam, 8

Spermicide, 88*t*

Stomach pain, 136

Stretch marks, 107

Sugaring, 30*t*

Suicide, 128–129

Syphilis, 82

T

Tampons, 47, 132–134

Tanner staging: breast development, 18*t*; public hair, 29*t*

Teratoma, 66

Terminal hair, 28, 34

Tetanus-diphtheria-pertussis (Tdap) booster, 99–100

Thyroid gland, 14

Thyroid stimulating hormone (TSH), 16

Torsion, ovarian, 71

Treponema pallidum, 82

Trichomonas vaginalis, 82

Trichomoniasis, 82

Trimming, 30*t*

Tuberculosis, 57

Turner syndrome, 50

Tweezing, 30*t*

U

Ulcers, vulvar, 63–64

Urethra, 12

Urethral diverticulum, 122

Urethral prolapse, 122; and vulvovaginitis, 61

Urethritis, 121

Urethrocele. *See* Urethral prolapse

www.ingramcontent.com/pod-product-compliance
Lightning Source LLC
Chambersburg PA
CBHW030109300326
41934CB00034B/663